A WHOLE
NEW WAY
TO EAT

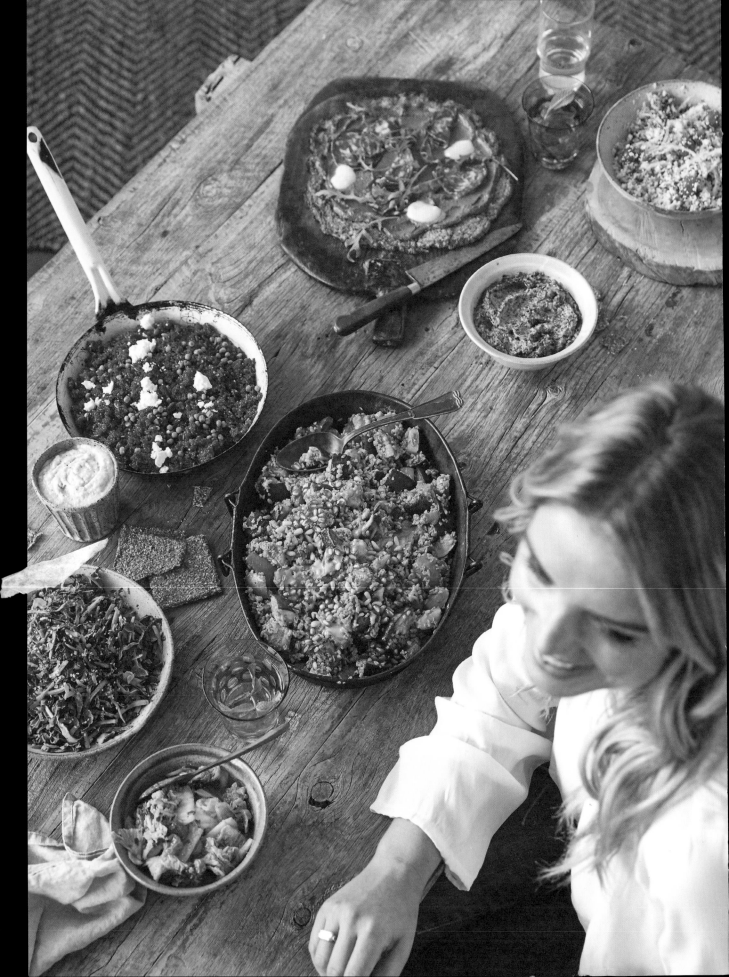

A WHOLE NEW WAY TO EAT

135+ FEEL-GOOD RECIPES
FROM **ABOUT LIFE**

———————

Vladia Cobrdova

MURDOCH BOOKS
SYDNEY · LONDON

FOREWORD

As you can imagine, my sister Tammie Phillips and I have strong ideas about food, but it hasn't always been such a huge part of our lives. We both once had corporate jobs that involved a lot of travel, jet lag, and food choices based on convenience. I think we knew our bodies needed to be fuelled but we didn't really understand how to get the best from what we ate.

As part of our extensive travels, we both lived in Japan for a while and loved the delicious diet there. I think that was when we first started to genuinely comprehend the relationship between nutritious food and longevity and quality of life. We also experienced the relatively new concept of the wholefood store and started thinking about how we could take these ideas back to Australia, not just as a café but as a whole new way of eating, a genuine alternative to the traditional supermarkets.

Not many people realise this, but About Life has been around since 1996, so we're no free-range spring chickens. It started off as a hundred-square-metre juice bar and café with a few shelves of natural groceries, situated just across the road from where our thriving Rozelle store is today. The founding principle of About Life has never changed: no food complexity, just simplicity and goodness. Everything we have built stems from this core belief and is the guiding principle in all our decisions; about the people we work with, the suppliers we choose and the way we market

ourselves. As the concept has grown, our interests have expanded to encompass a range of environmental and social issues and the range of products we offer reflects that.

In 2003, the fabulously talented, smart and creative Vladia Cobrdova entered the About Life story. We could not have found a person more attuned to our food philosophy. Vladia is the inspirational Wellness Ambassador for the company. You'll find many of the recipes in this book being cooked in the About Life kitchens, and the company would not be the pioneer of healthy food that it is today without her expertise and energy.

Vladia's food philosophy focuses on the importance of using the best possible natural ingredients, free from chemicals, and in tune with the balance of your body and with the seasons. She loves the flavours of naturally grown vegies, such as the simple pleasure of a sun-ripened tomato eaten with a pinch of salt. The recipes in this book are the culmination of years of knowledge, combining ingredients to create the perfect balance of health, nutrition and taste.

'Food as medicine' remains one of the cornerstones of the About Life philosophy, and Vladia's recipes will put a smile on your face and a spring in your step. But these dishes are also about the joy of sitting around the table with your loved ones, sharing satisfyingly delicious food.

Jodie Stewart

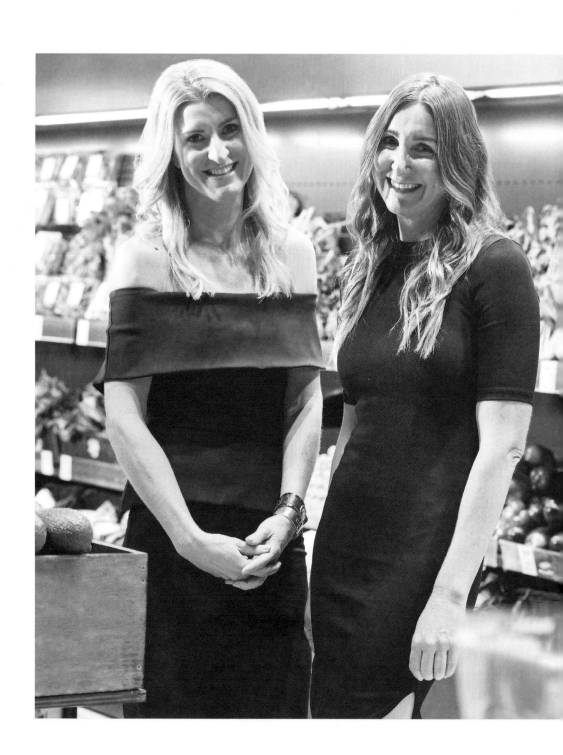

CONTENTS

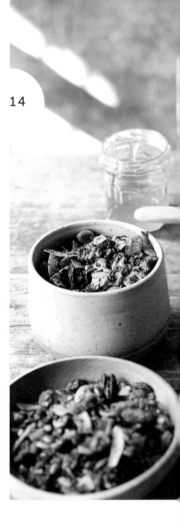

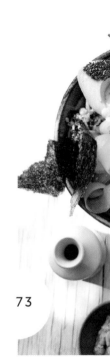

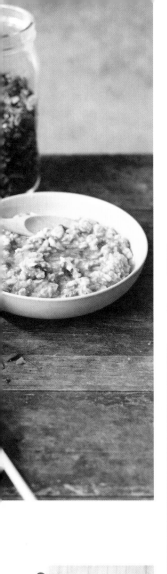

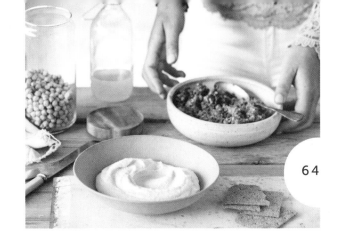

64

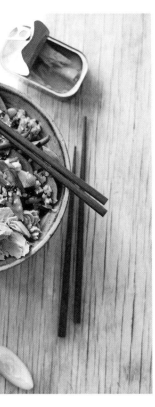

149

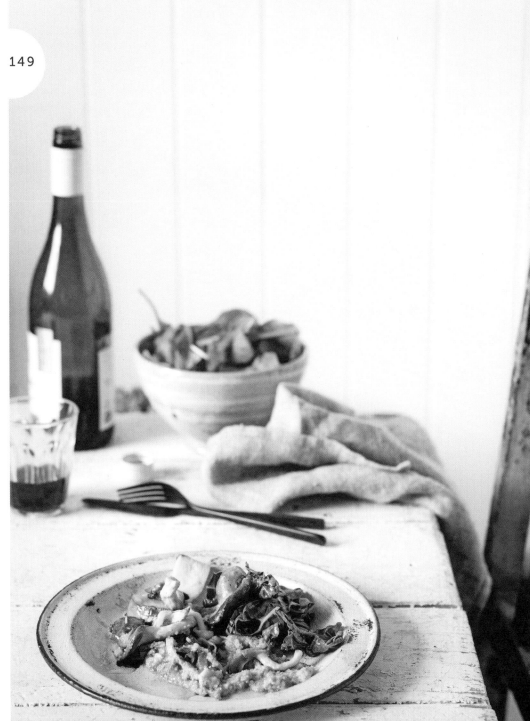

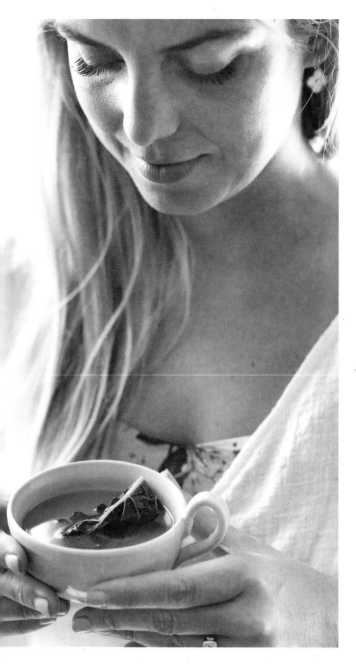

INTRODUCTION

Welcome to a whole new way to eat! This is a collection of natural, real recipes that your body will love, from your tastebuds to your gut. Everyone is welcome at the table with this way of eating, whether you're looking for inspirational recipes that are vegan, paleo or vegetarian, or simply after truly delicious food that just happens to be good for you.

At the wholefoods grocery store About Life, I develop recipes for the cafés and takeaway sections, and ready-made meals that showcase delicious local produce prepared in a way that surprises people by how healthy it is. My hope is that people can relax and be happy about what they put on their plate, recognising the effort that producers of top-quality chemical-free ingredients put in to bring you your food.

Where I grew up, in communist Czechoslovakia, the kitchen was the smallest room in the house but it was where the whole family gathered, busying ourselves preparing food, mingling and talking loudly to each other all the while. Food and its preparation was a joy – a family affair with plenty of laughter and experimentation. There was never a sense of some foods being bad or others being good.

Living in Australia now, I'm blown away by the range of ingredients that are available – it still astonishes me that there is so much variety. To me, each season has a unique smell: mangoes and cherries in summer; pears and plums in autumn; cauliflower and broccoli

EACH SEASON HAS A UNIQUE SMELL: MANGO AND CHERRY IN SUMMER; PEARS AND PLUMS IN AUTUMN; BROCCOLI AND CAULIFLOWER IN WINTER; FENNEL AND ASPARAGUS IN SPRING.

in winter; asparagus and fennel in spring. It's easy to eat seasonally, and it's become the cornerstone of my food philosophy.

But living here I am also amazed by the fact that so many of us are developing fears and obsessions about the very food we loved as children.

Since when did bread become evil? Sure, common supermarket bread – with all its additives and hidden ingredients – isn't great for you, but real fermented sourdough and rye breads are basic foods that deserve a place in our daily lives.

And why is dairy suddenly on the nose for so many? Real-deal dairy foods – that come from happy cows, sheep or goats – are so nourishing for us. The most frequently used product in my home kitchen surely must be yoghurt: I include it as an ingredient in or as an accompaniment to nearly everything I cook.

And don't get me started on fruit! I just don't understand why so many people are afraid of what I think of as nature's sweets. Have you ever eaten a chemical-free locally grown cherry tomato? They taste like confectionery produced by the land to be enjoyed seasonally. But of course you'll only get this taste if you eat them when they are naturally ripe and in season. Eating according to the seasons is doubly beneficial: you eat the food when it is most delicious and the best quality, and you are supporting local farmers and the environment.

The next step in respecting the work that goes into growing and producing your food is to try to use the whole food, wasting as little as possible. In some of my recipes you'll see I use the tops of beetroots, kale stalks and the outer leaves of cauliflower, which are usually discarded. Sometimes it's about having a rethink. What nutritious part of the vegetable or the animal are you throwing out because you've been brought up to think of it as waste? Could you use it for a simple broth or another dish with just a little bit of creativity?

The dishes in this book cover every occasion – for when you only have 10 minutes to prepare a nutritious snack to keep the energy levels up and the stress levels down, or for creating a meal to impress your guests. Perhaps you want to experience the sense of achievement you get from baking bread and serving it with lashings of good quality local butter. My hope is that by sharing these recipes, I can pass on some of the enjoyment and satisfaction that cooking has given my family and me, and that it gives me each day at About Life.

Vladia Cobrdova

BREAKFAST

+ VEGETARIAN
+ VEGAN
+ GLUTEN-FREE
+ DAIRY-FREE

PREP TIME:
*10 minutes,
plus 1 hour chilling*

COOKING TIME:
5 minutes

CACAO QUINOA BREAKFAST BOWL

*Who says you can't have chocolate for breakfast?
This bowl is delicious and filling: a source of
protein, carbs, antioxidants and more!*

SERVES 2

*370 g (13 oz/2 cups) cooked quinoa
(see note on page 12)*
*500 ml (17 fl oz/2 cups) tinned
coconut milk*
2 tablespoons cacao powder
2 tablespoons pure maple syrup
2 teaspoons ground cinnamon
2 tablespoons shredded coconut
70 g (2½ oz) blueberries
2 bananas, sliced
*2 tablespoons chopped
raw hazelnuts*

Put the quinoa and coconut milk in a saucepan and stir over medium heat for 2–3 minutes until heated through. Stir in the cacao powder, maple syrup and cinnamon and cook for another 2 minutes or until warmed through. Remove from the heat. Spoon into a bowl or jar, cover and refrigerate for 1 hour or until chilled.

To serve, divide the mixture between two bowls, then scatter with the remaining ingredients.

+ **NOTE** Tinned coconut milk is a marvellous dairy substitute. It is creamy and a little on the sweet side.

+ VEGETARIAN
+ VEGAN
+ GLUTEN-FREE
+ DAIRY-FREE

PREP TIME:
5 minutes

COOKING TIME:
5 minutes

COCONUT TURMERIC QUINOA PORRIDGE

This breakfast dish can also lend itself to being served as a side dish: it's more of a savoury porridge than a sweet one.

SERVES 2

370 g (13 oz/2 cups) cooked quinoa
    (see note)
375 ml (13 fl oz/1½ cups) tinned
    coconut milk
1 teaspoon ground turmeric
1 pinch cayenne pepper
¼ teaspoon pink Himalayan salt
2 tablespoons pepitas (pumpkin
    seeds)
2 tablespoons shredded coconut
Fruit and yoghurt, to serve

Combine all of the ingredients, except the pepitas and shredded coconut, in a saucepan and stir over medium heat until the mixture comes to the boil. Simmer for 3 minutes or until the creamy mixture starts to thicken, then remove from the heat. Divide the porridge between two bowls, scatter with the pepitas and shredded coconut and serve immediately with fruit and yoghurt.

+ **NOTE** Quinoa is a super grain that is very high in protein and fibre as well as being gluten free. When soaked overnight it is easier to digest. To make 370 g (13 oz/2 cups) of cooked quinoa, soak 135 g (4¾ oz/⅔ cup) of quinoa overnight in a large bowl of water. Drain and rinse well under cold running water to flush away the soapy residue (saponins). Put it in a saucepan with 330 ml (11¼ fl oz/1⅓ cups) of water, bring to the boil over high heat, then reduce the heat to as low as possible and simmer for 10 minutes or until the liquid is absorbed and the quinoa is soft.

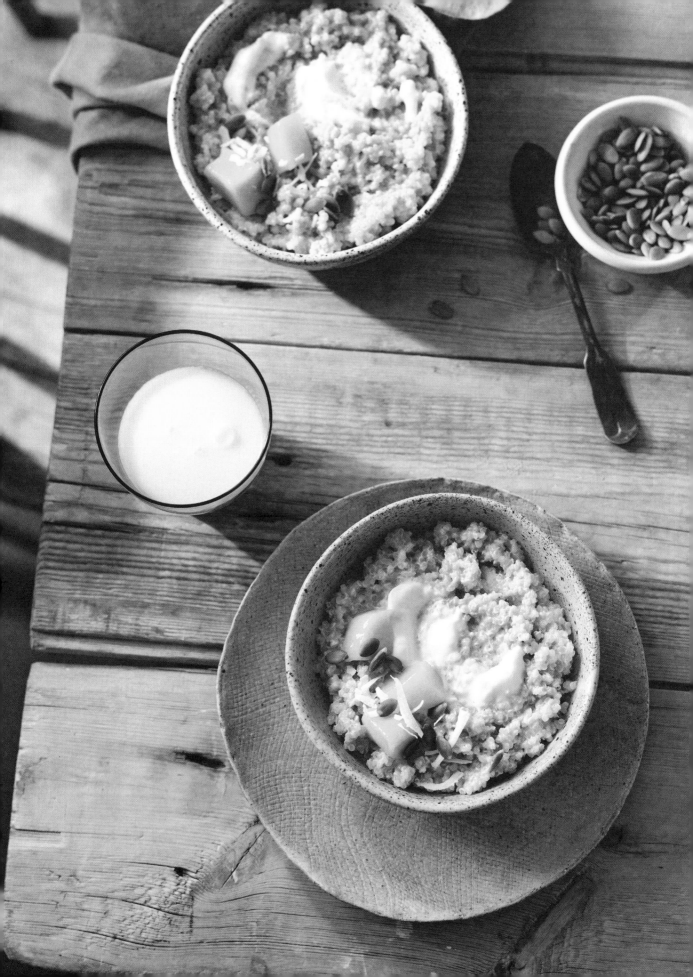

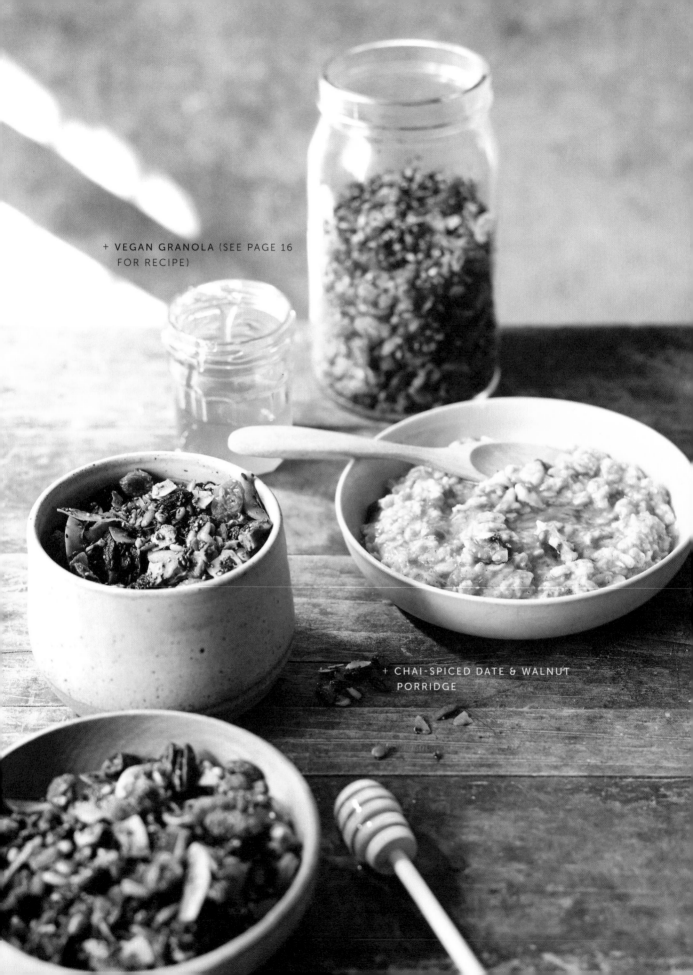

+ VEGAN GRANOLA (SEE PAGE 16 FOR RECIPE)

+ CHAI-SPICED DATE & WALNUT PORRIDGE

+ VEGETARIAN
+ VEGAN
+ GLUTEN-FREE
+ DAIRY-FREE

PREP TIME:
10 minutes

COOKING TIME:
10 minutes

CHAI-SPICED DATE & WALNUT PORRIDGE

This nurturing bowl of warming spices is a satisfying way to start your day.

SERVES 4

200 g (7 oz/2 cups) rolled (porridge) oats
1 tablespoon finely grated ginger
2 teaspoons ground cinnamon
85 g (3 oz/½ cup) pitted dates, chopped
4 star anise
½ teaspoon ground cloves
Zest and juice of 1 orange
45 g (1½ oz) toasted walnuts, chopped
2 tablespoons raw honey

Put the oats in a saucepan with 750 ml (26 fl oz/3 cups) of water and cook over medium heat, stirring occasionally, for 5 minutes or until the oats start to become creamy. Add the ginger, cinnamon, dates, star anise and cloves and cook for another 3 minutes or until the water starts to evaporate and the oats are creamy. Add the orange zest and juice and stir for 2 minutes or until well heated through. Remove the star anise and discard. Divide the porridge between two bowls, scatter the walnuts over and drizzle with the honey, then serve immediately.

+ **NOTE** Cinnamon is one of my favourite spices. The taste of cinnamon for me is out of this world! It reminds me of my mum, because she always has coffee with cinnamon and I remember its beautiful aroma wafting through our kitchen. This aromatic spice is great for stimulating blood sugar levels. It also has an amazingly high count of antioxidants.

+ VEGETARIAN
+ VEGAN
+ GLUTEN-FREE
+ DAIRY-FREE
+ PALEO

PREP TIME:
10 minutes

COOKING TIME:
30 minutes

VEGAN GRANOLA

Making your own granola is so enjoyable and this recipe is a combination of all my favourite crunchy bits. It's not too sweet and pairs brilliantly with any breakfast dish or even as a salad topper.

MAKES 5–6 CUPS

75 g (2¾ oz/½ cup) pepitas
    (pumpkin seeds)
75 g (2¾ oz/½ cup) sunflower seeds
25 g (1 oz/¼ cup) LSA meal
    (linseed, sunflower seed and
    almond meal)
40 g (1½ oz/¼ cup) linseeds
    (flaxseeds)
65 g (2½ oz/1½ cups) coconut chips
65 g (2½ oz/½ cup) cacao nibs
90 g (3¼ oz/½ cup) chia seeds
55 g (2 oz/½ cup) coarsely
    chopped pecans
80 ml (2½ fl oz/⅓ cup) sweet
    almond oil
1½ tablespoons maple syrup
1¼ tablespoons Digestive Spice
    (see page 175)
½ teaspoon pink Himalayan salt
100 g (3½ oz/½ cup) Peruvian
    groundcherries (Inca berries)
60 g (2¼ oz/½ cup) goji berries
65 g (2½ oz/½ cup) white
    mulberries

Preheat the oven to 150°C (300°F). Line a large baking tray with baking paper and set aside.

Combine all of the ingredients, except the Peruvian groundcherries, goji berries and mulberries, in a large bowl and mix well. Spread over the prepared baking tray and bake, stirring regularly, for 30 minutes or until lightly toasted and golden. Remove from the oven and allow to cool on the tray.

Stir through the combined berries, then store in an airtight container for up to 4 weeks.

+ **NOTE** This vegan granola is gluten free, grain free and full of good fats to boost your brain ability in the morning. It's also low in fructose.

GOLDEN SAVOURY FRENCH TOAST

My mum used to make savoury French toast all the time when we were kids. Now I'm all grown up, I have added more sophisticated ingredients that nourish. I use real sourdough, which is an amazing bread. Sourdough has been fermented, which is why it is easier to digest. It is a traditional bread that my great-grandparents used to make.

SERVES 2

2 eggs
80 ml (2½ fl oz/⅓ cup) kefir
   (or use plain yoghurt)
1 teaspoon ground turmeric
Sea salt
2 sourdough bread slices
2 tablespoons olive oil
1 avocado, halved lengthways,
   skin and stone discarded
1 tablespoon chopped dill
1 tablespoon lemon juice
½ teaspoon cayenne pepper
2 smoked salmon slices
Lemon wedges, to serve

Whisk the eggs in a shallow bowl with the kefir, turmeric and a pinch of sea salt until well combined. Soak the bread in the egg mixture for 2 minutes on each side.

Heat the olive oil in a frying pan over medium heat and fry the soaked bread for 4 minutes on each side or until golden.

Meanwhile, mash the avocado with the dill, lemon juice, cayenne pepper and salt. Divide the French toast between two plates, top with the avocado and smoked salmon and serve with lemon wedges.

+ **NOTE** Turmeric not only adds a lovely golden colour, it also has anti-inflammatory properties. I often add it to my broths and smoothies.

+ VEGETARIAN
+ VEGAN
+ DAIRY-FREE

PREP TIME:
15 minutes

COOKING TIME:
Nil

BREAKFAST ORANGE & ALMOND COUSCOUS

Light and full of cinnamon flavour, this dish is great for breakfast served with yoghurt, but also as a salad on its own. It makes a great accompaniment to lamb or chicken, too.

SERVES 2

190 g (6¾ oz/1 cup) couscous
2 teaspoons mixed spice,
    such as Beat Sugar Cravings
    (see page 175)
1 teaspoon melted coconut oil
375 ml (13 fl oz/1½ cups) boiling
    water
Juice of 1 orange
1 teaspoon orange zest
45 g (1½ oz/¼ cup) raisins
40 g (1½ oz/¼ cup) toasted
    almond kernels, chopped
40 g (1½ oz/¼ cup) dried
    cranberries
15 g (½ oz/¼ cup) chopped
    mint leaves
Yoghurt, to serve

Put the couscous in a heatproof bowl and stir the mixed spice and coconut oil through. Pour the boiling water over, stir to combine, then cover and set aside for 10 minutes or until all the liquid has been absorbed. Using a fork, fluff the couscous to separate the grains, then stir in the orange juice and zest, raisins, almonds and cranberries. Scatter with the mint and serve with yoghurt.

————

+ **NOTE** Oranges contain vitamin C; couscous is an excellent source of vegetarian protein as well as a good source of fibre.

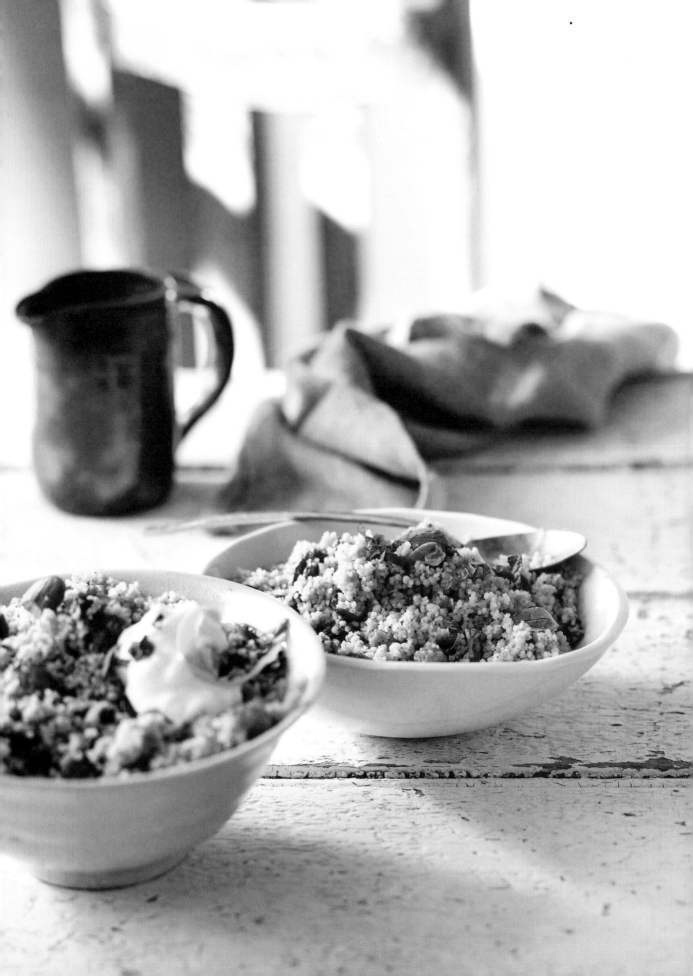

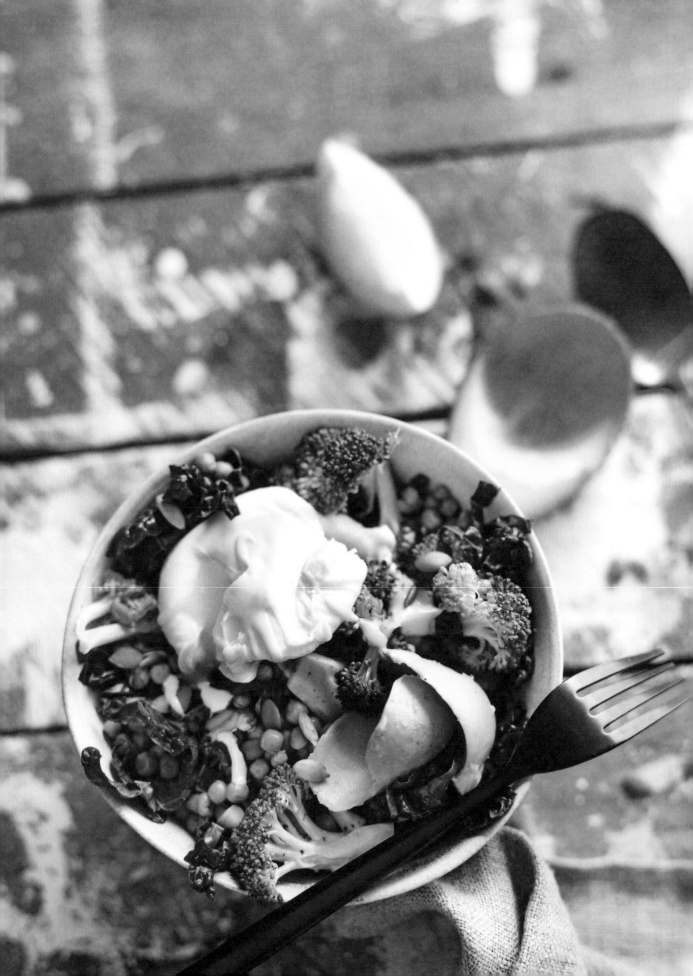

+ VEGETARIAN
+ GLUTEN-FREE
+ DAIRY-FREE
+ PALEO

PREP TIME:
10 minutes

COOKING TIME:
10 minutes

GREEN BREKKIE BOWL

Salads for breakfast fill you up and give a good boost of minerals and vitamins to get you ready for the long day ahead.

SERVES 2

1 teaspoon coconut oil
180 g (6¼ oz) broccoli, cut into small florets (about 3 cups)
2 large kale leaves, thinly sliced, stalks removed (about 2 cups)
140 g (5 oz/1 cup) frozen peas
2 tablespoons lemon juice
2 eggs
1 tablespoon apple cider vinegar
2 tablespoons pepitas (pumpkin seeds)
1 avocado, halved lengthways, skin and stone discarded, thinly sliced
Lemon wedges, to serve

TURMERIC TAHINI DRESSING
135 g (4¾ oz/½ cup) tahini
Juice of ½ lemon
1 teaspoon salt
60 ml (2 fl oz/¼ cup) olive oil
2 teaspoons ground turmeric

Heat the coconut oil in a frying pan over medium heat, add the broccoli, kale and peas and cook for 4 minutes or until the broccoli is tender. Add the lemon juice, season with salt and freshly ground black pepper to taste and remove from the heat.

Meanwhile, to poach the eggs, fill a deep-sided frying pan with water to 8 cm (3¼ inches) deep. Add the vinegar and bring to the boil over medium heat. Crack the eggs into small separate bowls, taking care not to break the yolks. Using a wooden spoon, stir the water clockwise to create a whirlpool. Carefully tip the eggs, one at a time, into the centre of the whirlpool, then skim any foam from the top of the water. Cook gently for 3 minutes or until cooked to your liking; the water should only just bubble, not boil. Remove the eggs with a slotted spoon and pat dry briefly on a clean tea towel (dish towel).

To make the dressing, combine all of the ingredients in a small bowl. Add 60 ml (2 fl oz/¼ cup) of water and use a fork to combine well.

To serve, divide the greens between two plates, top with the poached eggs, pepitas and avocado. Drizzle with a generous amount of the turmeric tahini dressing and serve with lemon wedges.

PREP TIME:
10 minutes

COOKING TIME:
10 minutes

EGG NOURISHMENT

This is a bestselling dish in our cafés: we change menus seasonally, but I would not dare touch this one. People from all over ask for the recipe for this tasty creation — so delicious and creamy, and good to eat at any time of day — so we've included it again in this book. It's a winner!

SERVES 2 AS A MAIN OR 4 AS A SIDE

1 tablespoon olive oil
1 red (Spanish) onion, finely
    chopped
370 g (13 oz/2 cups) cooked quinoa
    (see note on page 12)
4 eggs
4 tablespoons basil pesto (home-
    made or ready-made is fine)
160 g (5¾ oz) cherry tomatoes,
    halved
50 g (1¾ oz/2 cups) finely chopped
    cavolo nero or kale leaves,
    stalks removed
1 teaspoon each salt and freshly
    ground black pepper
1 tablespoon linseeds (flaxseeds)
Lemon wedges, to serve

Heat the olive oil in a large frying pan over medium heat. Add the onion and stir for 3–4 minutes until golden. Add the cooked quinoa and stir until heated through. Whisk the eggs, add to the pan and stir through. Add the pesto and stir through for 1 minute. Add the cherry tomatoes, cavolo nero, salt and pepper and mix for another minute. Remove from the heat and divide between two bowls. Sprinkle with linseeds and serve immediately with lemon wedges.

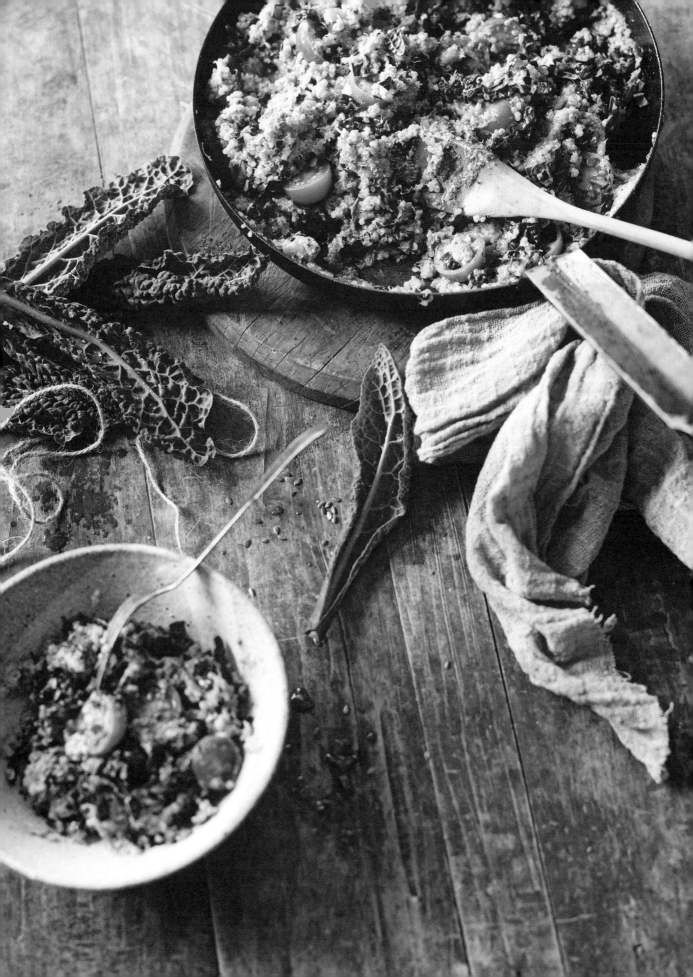

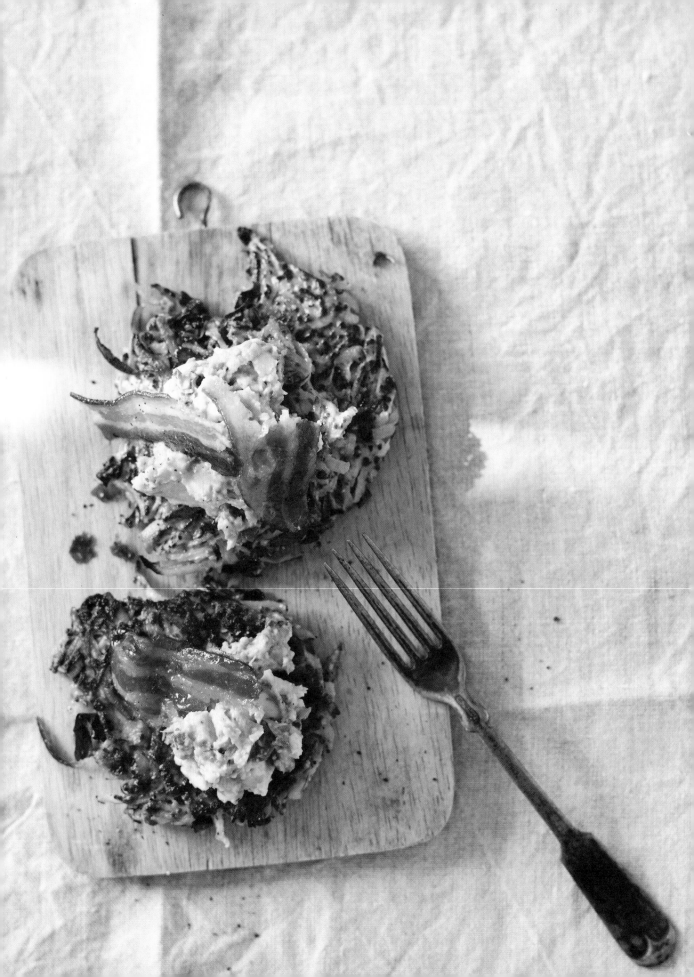

PREP TIME:
20 minutes

COOKING TIME:
25 minutes

KOHLRABI & SWEET POTATO ROSTI WITH MAPLE BACON AND LIME AVOCADO

My mum used to make this recipe at home, minus the bacon and avocado. The first time I tasted avocado was when I arrived in Australia, and it's now one of my favourite ingredients, as it's so nutritious and makes everything taste luscious.

SERVES 4 (MAKES 12)

4 eggs
90 g (3¼ oz/½ cup) chia seeds
175 g (6 oz/about ½) kohlrabi,
    peeled and grated
260 g (9¼ oz/about ½ large)
    sweet potato, grated
2 spring onions (scallions),
    thinly sliced
2 kale leaves, finely chopped,
    stalks removed (about 2 cups)
4 bacon slices, cut into thirds
60 ml (2 fl oz/¼ cup) pure
    maple syrup
2 avocados, halved lengthways,
    skin and stones discarded
Zest and juice of 1 lime
2 tablespoons chopped mint leaves
2 tablespoons ghee

Preheat the oven to 160°C (315°F).

To make the rosti mixture, put the eggs, chia seeds, kohlrabi, sweet potato, spring onions and kale in a large bowl and stir to combine well. Stand for 10 minutes to allow the chia seeds to absorb the moisture. Season with salt and freshly ground black pepper.

Meanwhile, lay the bacon on a baking tray lined with baking paper and brush both sides with the maple syrup. Bake for 15 minutes or until crisp.

Coarsely mash the avocado flesh with the lime zest and juice and the mint, season with salt and freshly ground black pepper, then set aside. (I like my avocado mash chunky so you can feel the texture.)

Heat the ghee in a large frying pan over high heat. Working in batches, drop heaped tablespoons of the rosti mixture into the pan and cook for 4 minutes on each side or until golden, then drain on paper towel. Divide the rostis between four serving plates, top with avo mash and bacon and serve immediately.

RAINBOW TURMERIC SCRAMBLED EGGS

I always try to find a way to incorporate more vegies into my diet, especially at breakfast time. As well as this recipe, I also love scrambled eggs with thyme, kale and basil, or beetroot (beets), spinach and chives.

SERVES 2

1 carrot, roughly chopped
1 teaspoon chopped fresh ginger
1 teaspoon ground turmeric
4 eggs
¼ teaspoon pink Himalayan salt
2 teaspoons coconut oil

Put the carrot, ginger and turmeric in a high-speed blender with 60 ml (2 fl oz/¼ cup) of water and process to combine.

Lightly beat the eggs in a bowl with the salt, then whisk in the carrot mixture until well combined.

Heat the coconut oil in a frying pan over low heat. Add the egg mixture and cook, stirring gently for 5–7 minutes until cooked to your liking. Serve immediately, perhaps with Purple Seeded Bread (see page 31).

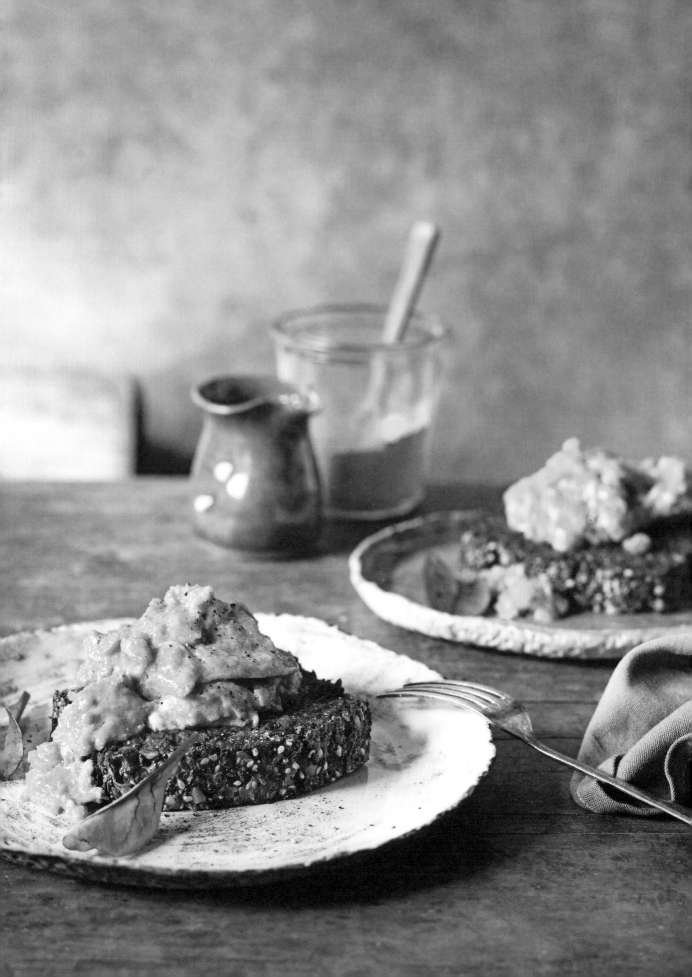

+ GLUTEN-FREE
+ DAIRY-FREE
+ PALEO

PREP TIME:
10 minutes

COOKING TIME:
15 minutes

MUSCLE BREKKIE BOWL

This recipe is great fuel for breakfast and pairs the taste of sweet potato with the saltiness of bacon.

SERVES 2

150 g (5½ oz) bacon, chopped
2 eggs
500 g (1 lb 2 oz/2 cups) Spicy
    Cinnamon Sweet Potato Mash
    (see page 193)
90 g (3¼ oz/2 cups) baby spinach
    leaves
2 large kale leaves, thinly sliced,
    stalks removed, (about 2 cups)
1 teaspoon dried chilli flakes
2 tablespoons chopped coriander
    (cilantro) leaves
Lemon wedges, to serve

Cook the bacon in a nonstick frying pan over high heat until golden. Drain on paper towel, then return the pan to medium heat and fry the eggs until cooked to your liking.

Meanwhile, put the sweet potato mash in a saucepan and stir over medium heat until warmed through, then fold in the spinach and kale. Stir for 2 minutes or until the spinach starts to wilt, then remove from the heat.

To serve, divide the mash mixture between two bowls and top with the bacon and eggs. Scatter with the chilli flakes and coriander leaves and serve with lemon wedges.

+ **NOTE** When choosing bacon, I recommend choosing the lowest nitrate option.

+ VEGETARIAN
+ VEGAN
+ GLUTEN-FREE
+ DAIRY-FREE

PREP TIME:
5 minutes

COOKING TIME:
10 minutes

CHIA'ZY AVOCADO TOAST

This is a bestseller in our cafés. Everyone goes crazy for this simple but delicious dish, which is suitable for breakfast or lunch, and we couldn't resist repeating the recipe in this book. Serve it with sourdough or rye bread, or try my Purple Seeded Bread (see page 31).

SERVES 2

1 tablespoon coconut oil
1 small red (Spanish) onion, finely chopped
160 g (5¾ oz) cherry tomatoes, halved
¼ teaspoon each salt and freshly ground black pepper
2 bread slices
4 tablespoons Chia'zy Avocado Dip (see page 62)
2 teaspoons black chia seeds
2 tablespoons coriander (cilantro) leaves
Lemon wedges, to serve

Heat the coconut oil in a frying pan over medium heat. Add the onion and cook for 3 minutes or until translucent. Add the tomatoes, salt and pepper and cook for 5 minutes or until the tomatoes are a little mushy, then remove from the heat.

Meanwhile, toast the bread. Spread each slice with the avocado dip, then top with the hot tomato mixture. Scatter the chia seeds and coriander leaves over and serve with lemon wedges.

+ **NOTE** What is the difference between black and white chia seeds? Nutritionally, they are more or less the same. I like to choose a contrasting colour to give visual interest to a dish.

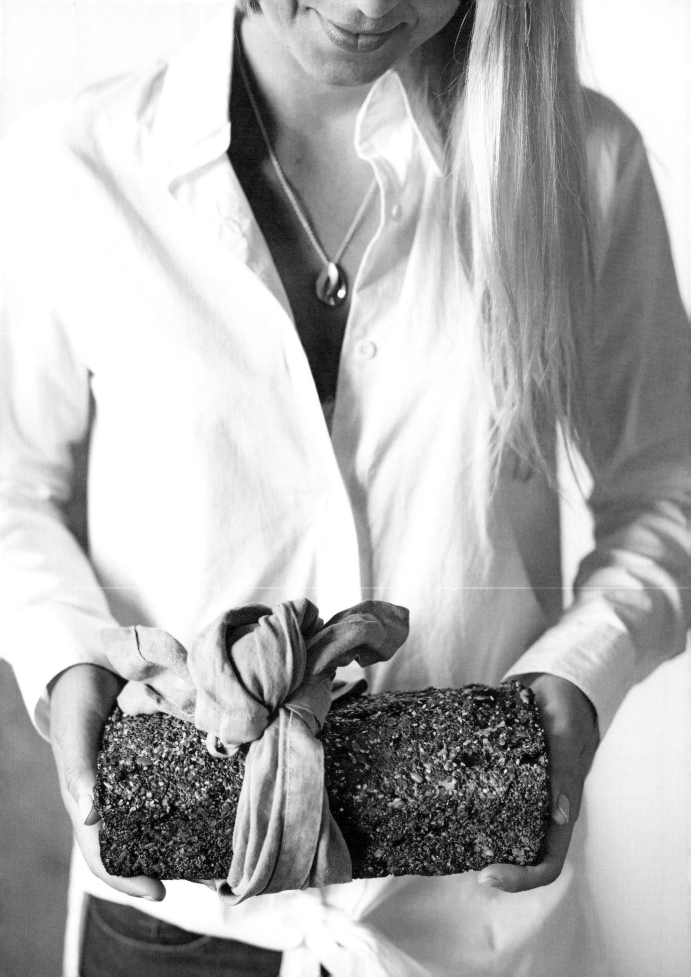

+ VEGETARIAN
+ GLUTEN-FREE
+ PALEO

PREP TIME:
20 minutes, plus overnight standing

COOKING TIME:
2¼ hours

PURPLE SEEDED BREAD

Purple is the new black: more colour in your food means more nutrients. I am always pleased with this bread when it comes out of the oven: the purple colour looks amazing and it tastes so good!

MAKES 1 LOAF

1 purple sweet potato, about
    400 g (14 oz), scrubbed and
    quartered lengthways
4 purple carrots, scrubbed
    and halved
85 g (3 oz/½ cup) linseeds
    (flaxseeds)
90 g (3¼ oz/½ cup) chia seeds
50 g (1¾ oz/½ cup) LSA meal
    (linseed, sunflower seed and
    almond meal)
75 g (2¾ oz/½ cup) sesame seeds
75 g (2¾ oz/½ cup) pepitas
    (pumpkin seeds)
75 g (2¾ oz/½ cup) sunflower
    seeds
2 teaspoons salt
200 g (7 oz/1 cup) black quinoa
125 ml (4 fl oz/½ cup) kefir
    (or use plain yoghurt)
5 eggs, lightly beaten
1 tablespoon mustard oil
1½ tablespoons dijon mustard
1 tablespoon finely chopped
    rosemary

Preheat the oven to 170°C (325°F).

Lay the sweet potato and carrots on a lightly greased baking tray and bake for 45 minutes or until very tender. Allow to cool, then mash together in a large mixing bowl. Add all of the remaining ingredients and combine well, then cover and refrigerate overnight.

The following day, preheat the oven to 160°C (315°F). Lightly grease a 25 x 10 cm (10 x 4 inch) loaf (bar) tin and line the base and sides with baking paper.

Pour the chilled mixture into the prepared tin and bake for 1½ hours or until a skewer inserted in the centre comes out clean. Stand in the tin until cool. The bread will keep for up to 1 week wrapped tightly in plastic wrap in the fridge.

+ **NOTE** This bread is nutrient dense. Adding kefir aids digestion, meaning it's great for our guts. If you can't find purple carrots and purple sweet potatoes you can use golden carrots and golden sweet potatoes; and if you like the purple colour you can substitute beetroot (beets) for the carrots.

+ VEGETARIAN
+ GLUTEN-FREE
+ PALEO

PREP TIME:
20 minutes

COOKING TIME:
40 minutes

HIGH-PROTEIN MUFFINS

*Deliciously low carb, gluten free and loaded
with protein, these muffins are the perfect
midmorning snack.*

MAKES 6 LARGE MUFFINS

450 g (1 lb/about 1 large) sweet
    potato, peeled
6 eggs
150 ml (5 fl oz) pure maple syrup
300 g (10½ oz) almond butter
1 banana, sliced
130 g (4½ oz/1 cup) coconut flour
1 tablespoon baking powder
3 teaspoons bicarbonate of soda
    (baking soda)
1 tablespoon ground cinnamon
1 teaspoon salt
1 tablespoon protein powder
60 g (2¼ oz) feta cheese, crumbled
40 g (1½ oz/¼ cup) pepitas
    (pumpkin seeds)

Preheat the oven to 160°C (315°F). Insert paper cases into
the holes of a 6-hole giant muffin tin.

Finely grate 140 g (5 oz) of the sweet potato and coarsely
chop the remainder. Put the chopped sweet potato into
a saucepan, cover with cold water and bring to the boil
over high heat. Cook for 7 minutes or until very tender,
then drain and mash until smooth.

Whisk the eggs and maple syrup together in a large
bowl. Add the mashed sweet potato, almond butter,
sliced banana and 40 g (1½ oz) of the raw grated sweet
potato and stir to combine well.

Sift the coconut flour, baking powder, bicarbonate of
soda, cinnamon, salt and protein powder into a bowl.
Add to the egg mixture and stir to combine. Spoon the
mixture into the paper cases in the muffin holes, then
top with the remaining grated sweet potato. Scatter with
the feta cheese and pepitas, then bake for 30 minutes or
until a skewer inserted into the centre comes out clean.

+ **NOTE** Maple syrup is a valuable sweetener that is
    less processed than granulated sugar. Using it won't
    give you a spike in your blood sugar levels. It also
    contains antioxidants and minerals.

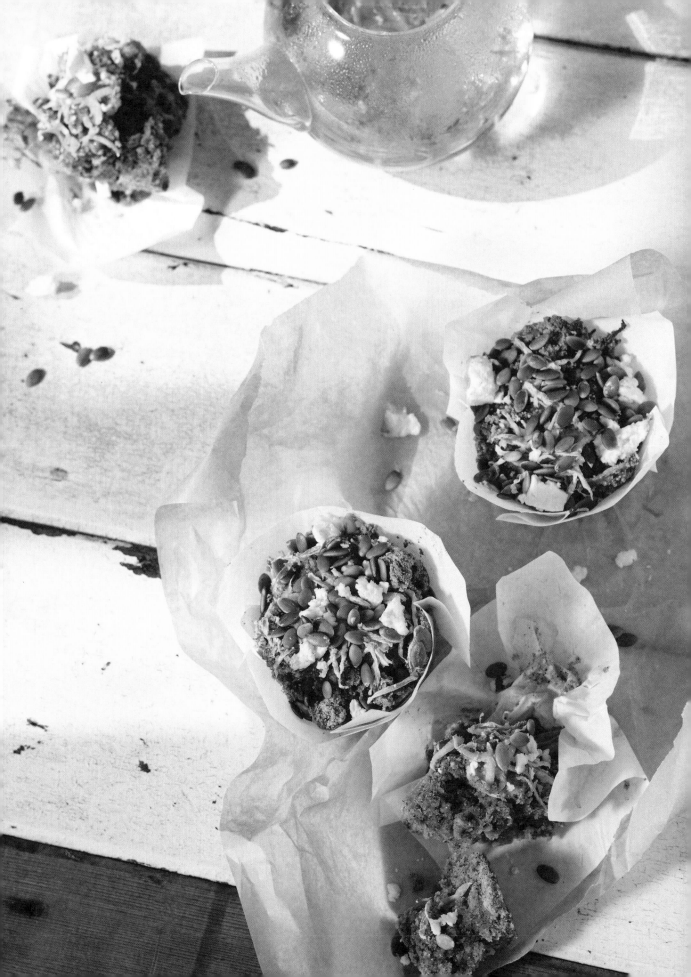

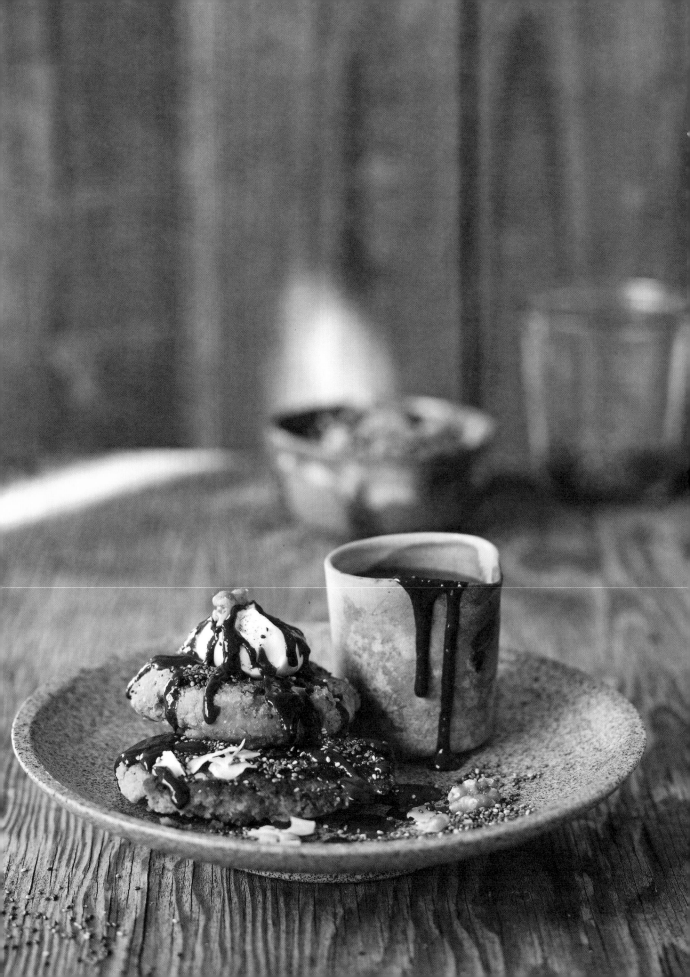

+ VEGETARIAN
+ GLUTEN-FREE
+ DAIRY-FREE
+ PALEO

PREP TIME:
15 minutes

COOKING TIME:
1 hour 10 minutes

SWEET POTATO PANCAKES

This breakfast dish is very popular in our cafés. It's the perfect combo of sweet potatoes and cacao that we serve with coconut yoghurt, but you can use cow's milk yoghurt too.

SERVES 2

1 small sweet potato, about
    350 g (12 oz), scrubbed
1 banana
1 egg
2 tablespoons chia seeds,
    plus extra for sprinkling
50 g (1¾ oz) coconut flour
Coconut oil, for frying
Sliced banana, extra (optional)
95 g (3¼ oz/⅓ cup) coconut
    yoghurt
2 teaspoons ground cinnamon
Coconut flakes and toasted
    chopped walnuts, to serve

CACAO SAUCE
60 g (2¼ oz/½ cup) cacao powder
125 ml (4 fl oz/½ cup) coconut oil
50 g (1¾ oz/¼ cup) coconut sugar
1 tablespoon chia seeds

Preheat the oven to 160°C (315°F). Put the sweet potato on a baking tray and bake for 1 hour or until soft. Remove from the oven and allow to cool.

Meanwhile, to make the cacao sauce, combine all of the ingredients in a bowl and mix well to combine. You may need to slightly melt the coconut oil if it is very solid.

Peel the sweet potato, put the flesh in a bowl with the banana and mash until smooth. Add the egg, chia seeds and coconut flour and stir until well combined.

Heat some coconut oil in a large shallow frying pan over high heat. Scoop two-tablespoon dollops of the mixture into the pan and cook for 4 minutes on each side or until golden. Divide the pancakes between two plates, top with slices of banana (if using) and sprinkle with the cinnamon and extra chia seeds. Add a dollop of the yoghurt on top. Drizzle with the cacao sauce, then scatter the coconut flakes and toasted chopped walnuts over and serve immediately.

DRINKS

+ VEGETARIAN
+ VEGAN
+ GLUTEN-FREE
+ DAIRY-FREE

PREP TIME:
5 minutes

COOKING TIME:
Nil

GREEN BLAST

Delicious and refreshing, this juice mix may help energise your body and boost the oxygen supply to your bloodstream. I've included this juice as part of my detox regime over many years, so it's an old recipe but a good one.

SERVES 1

185 g (6½ oz/about ½ bunch) kale, stalks included, roughly chopped
240 g (8¾ oz/about ½ bunch) English spinach, ends trimmed, leaves and stems washed well, roughly chopped
3 cm (1¼ inch) piece ginger, unpeeled
2 celery stalks
1 Lebanese (short) cucumber
2 teaspoons liquid chlorophyll

Press all of the ingredients except the liquid chlorophyll through a juicer. Stir in the chlorophyll and serve immediately.

+ **NOTE** Kale is high in fibre and iron and low in kilojoules, making it a useful addition to your diet. Rich green liquid chlorophyll is a green powerhouse adding an extra boost of nutrients into your diet; it's said to be an effective detoxifier and good for longevity.

+ VEGETARIAN
+ VEGAN
+ GLUTEN-FREE
+ DAIRY-FREE
+ PALEO

PREP TIME:
5 minutes

COOKING TIME:
Nil

KICKSTART MORNING DRINK

*I love to have this cup first thing in the morning
to kickstart my metabolism. It's also great as an
afternoon slump pick-me-up, instead of coffee
or hot chocolate. It can also be served chilled.*

SERVES 1

2 teaspoons Cinnamon Five Spice
   (see page 174)
2 teaspoons finely grated ginger
Juice of 1 lemon
250 ml (9 fl oz/1 cup) hot water
1 tablespoon raw honey,
   or use vegan sweetener
1 pinch dried chilli flakes

Put all of the ingredients into a mug, stir to combine
well and enjoy.

———

+ **NOTE** Cinnamon Five Spice is a combination of
cinnamon, star anise, black pepper, fennel, cloves and
pink Himalayan salt. All these spices get you moving
in the morning; not only your body, but also your
digestive system and metabolism!

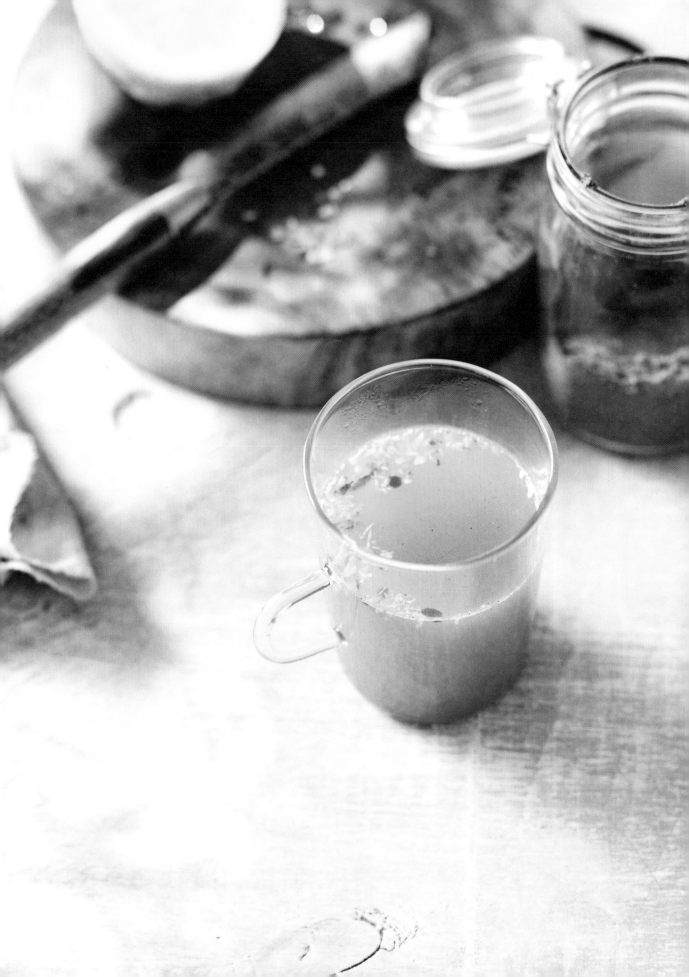

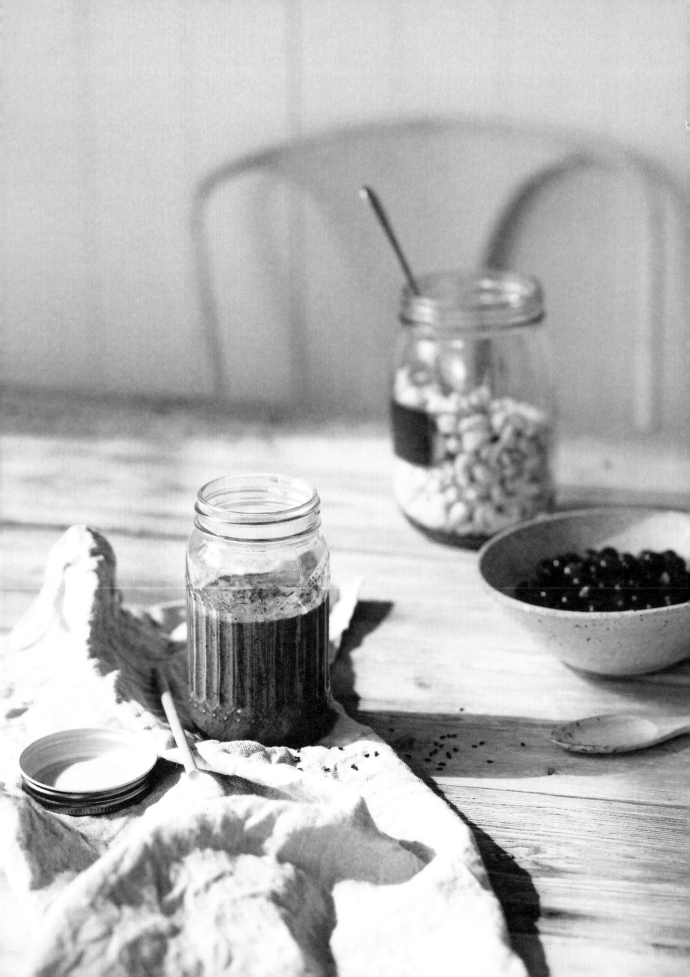

+ VEGETARIAN
+ VEGAN
+ GLUTEN-FREE
+ DAIRY-FREE

BLACK TAHINI SMOOTHIE

Sesame seeds are reputed to be a longevity food: an ancient staple. This velvety, luscious smoothie is my favourite when I feel like a sweet treat: it gets me going no matter what the time of day — morning or evening. It's a great breakfast and post work-out drink!

SERVES 1

155 g (5½ oz/1 cup) blueberries
2 dates, pitted
1 tablespoon protein powder
2 tablespoons black tahini
½ teaspoon ground cinnamon
50 g (1¾ oz/⅓ cup) raw cashews
375 ml (13 fl oz/1½ cups) coconut milk (dairy substitute)
6 ice cubes
1 teaspoon black sesame seeds

Blitz all of the ingredients, except the black sesame seeds, in a blender until a thin consistency is achieved. Sprinkle with the sesame seeds and serve immediately.

+ **NOTE** Black tahini is a source of plant-based calcium. It adds a creamy rich and nutty flavour to any dish or smoothie. You can use regular tahini if you prefer, or any nut butter.

KEFIR SMOOTHIE

Kefir is another longevity drink that is also an immunity builder. Kefir adds a range of good bacteria to your gut, which supports overall wellbeing. From your immune system to happiness: yes, I believe happiness is also built in the gut, so drink yourself happy with a range of friendly bacteria drinks such as kefir. Cheers!

SERVES 1

65 g (2½ oz) fresh or frozen
    baby peas
250 ml (9 fl oz/1 cup) kefir
45 g (1½ oz/1 cup) baby spinach
    leaves
1 fresh or frozen banana
125 ml (4 fl oz/½ cup) tinned
    coconut milk, plus extra
    to serve
1 teaspoon raw honey, plus extra
    to serve
6 mint leaves

Blitz all of the ingredients in a blender until a thick, smooth consistency is achieved. To serve, stir through a few drizzles of coconut milk and drizzle with honey.

+ **NOTE** Serve this smoothie in a bowl topped with your favourite crunchy granola or fruit.

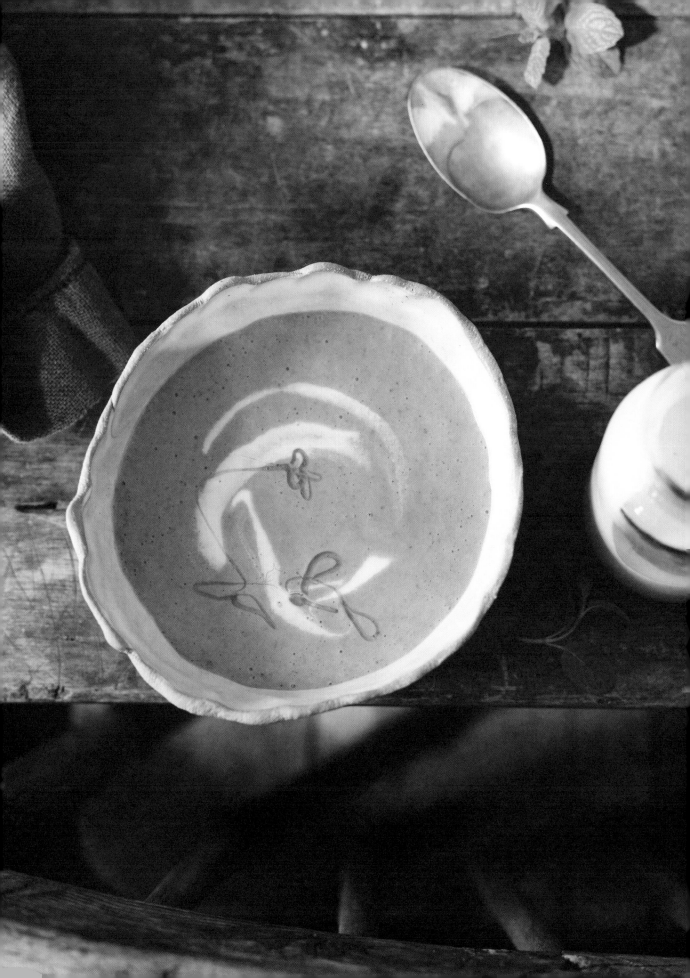

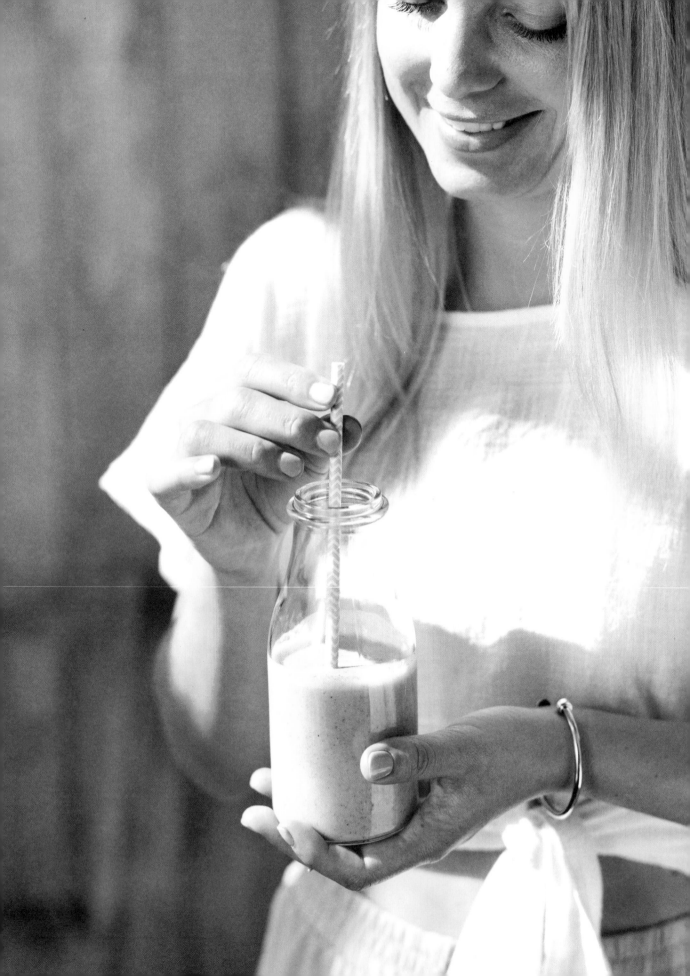

+ VEGETARIAN
+ VEGAN
+ GLUTEN-FREE
+ DAIRY-FREE

PREP TIME:
5 minutes

COOKING TIME:
Nil

SALTED ALMOND BUTTER SMOOTHIE

Almond butter is such a versatile spread and, luckily, it is also very nutritious. It's an effective way to add essential protein, vitamins and minerals to your diet. I often use it in smoothies like this: it adds a punch of protein and good fats. It's also delicious on morning toast and can be used in baking or as a porridge topping.

SERVES 1

1 banana
2 tablespoons crunchy almond
    butter
250 ml (9 fl oz/1 cup) coconut
    milk (dairy substitute)
125 ml (4 fl oz/½ cup) coconut
    water
1 tablespoon protein powder
½ teaspoon ground cinnamon
1 pinch pink Himalayan salt
6 ice cubes

Blitz all of the ingredients in a blender to a thick and creamy consistency. Serve immediately.

+ **NOTE** Have you tried almond butter dipping sauce? So easy! Just add coconut milk, tamari and a little water to thin out to a saucy consistency. Just like that, you have a dipping sauce to use for rice-paper rolls, veggie chips or even chicken. The best thing about it is that you know exactly what has gone into the sauce. Enjoy!

+ VEGETARIAN
+ VEGAN
+ GLUTEN-FREE
+ DAIRY-FREE

SILKY BAOBAB SMOOTHIE

Made from a native African fruit, baobab powder is very high in antioxidants (it has more antioxidants than acai berries, goji berries or blueberries) as well as magnesium and potassium. It's also low in sodium, sugar and kilojoules. It's a nutrition and fibre powerhouse for healthy digestion, reducing inflammation and supporting a healthy immune system.

SERVES 1

150 g (5½ oz/1 cup) fresh or frozen
  strawberries, hulled
1 peach, chopped
2 tablespoons LSA meal
  (linseed, sunflower seed
  and almond meal)
2 tablespoons silken tofu
1 tablespoon baobab powder
250 ml (9 fl oz/1 cup) almond
  milk
1 teaspoon raw honey,
  or use vegan sweetener
½ teaspoon bee pollen (optional)

Blitz all of the ingredients, except the bee pollen, in a blender until a thick consistency is achieved. Sprinkle with the bee pollen (if using) and serve immediately.

+ **NOTE** I love bee pollen: it comes in the form of crunchy sprinkles and it can be used as a topping on smoothie bowls, yoghurt and porridge or in smoothies. Bee pollen is the food of young bees and contains close to 50 per cent protein; it has almost all of the nutrients that your body needs. Although it's expensive, it's my choice of a wholefood multivitamin.

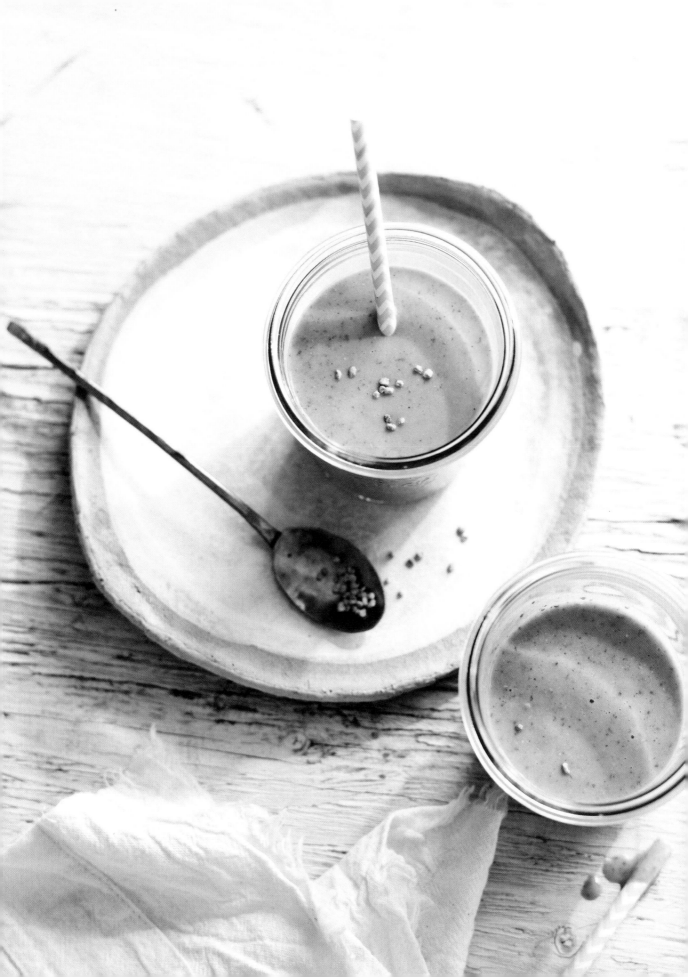

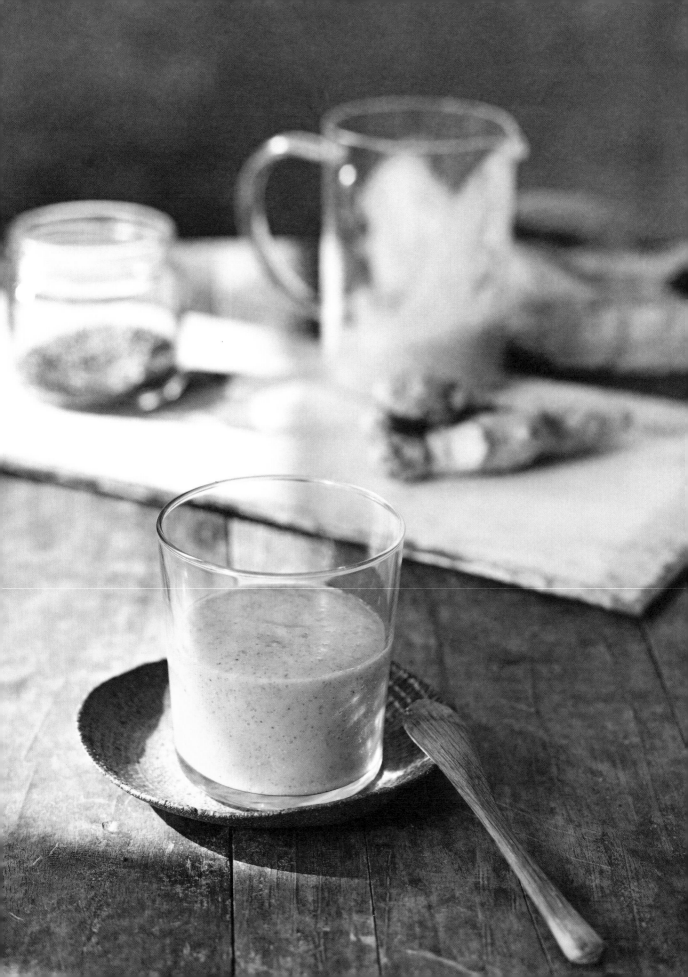

+ VEGETARIAN
+ VEGAN
+ GLUTEN-FREE
+ DAIRY-FREE
+ PALEO

PREP TIME:
5 minutes

COOKING TIME:
Nil

ZUCCHINI & MANGO SMOOTHIE

Having a smoothie for breakfast is a smart way to start the day. Zucchini and mango are a surprisingly tasty combination.

SERVES 1

100 g (3½ oz/1 cup) zucchini (courgette), ends trimmed, chopped
120 g (4¼ oz/½ cup) frozen chopped mango
1 teaspoon chia seeds
½ teaspoon finely chopped ginger
250 ml (9 fl oz/1 cup) coconut milk (dairy substitute)

Blitz all of the ingredients in a blender until a thick consistency is achieved. Serve immediately.

———

+ **NOTE** Mango: the smell of summer. This tropical fruit is good for your skin, both inside and out. Enjoy this nutritious smoothie to drink, or use it on your face as a refreshing mask!

+ VEGETARIAN
+ VEGAN
+ GLUTEN-FREE
+ DAIRY-FREE
+ PALEO

PREP TIME:
5 minutes

COOKING TIME:
Nil

TURMERIC GINGER LATTE

*Since we created this recipe at About Life a few
years ago, it has become one of our best sellers,
so it had to make its way into this book.
It's a fantastic substitute for coffee.*

SERVES 1

*3 cm (1¼ inch) piece ginger,
    unpeeled, grated
185 ml (6 fl oz/¾ cup) hot water
¼ teaspoon ground turmeric,
    plus extra to serve
250 ml (9 fl oz/1 cup) hot, frothy
    coconut milk (dairy substitute)*

Put the ginger and hot water in a small bowl and stand
for 3 minutes.

Strain the ginger water through a fine sieve into a latte
glass and discard the solids. Stir in the turmeric, then
top up the glass with the hot frothy coconut milk.
Sprinkle with a little extra ground turmeric and
serve immediately.

+ **NOTE** Turmeric and ginger: these potent herbs are
    botanically related to each other and are known
    remedies for gastrointestinal problems and
    inflammatory conditions. They are used to treat
    nausea, colds and other respiratory conditions and
    are believed to protect the brain from damage caused
    by Alzheimer's disease. This is one super cuppa.

+ VEGETARIAN
+ VEGAN
+ GLUTEN-FREE
+ DAIRY-FREE

PREP TIME:
5 minutes

COOKING TIME:
Nil

CAROB & MACA LATTE

Get grounded with this little beauty: I say it's powerful and down to earth. Carob is high in potassium, magnesium and protein; cayenne gets your body burning kilojoules; and maca is said to alleviate pain and cramps while it boosts energy, mood and general health.

SERVES 1

½ teaspoon carob powder
½ teaspoon maca powder
1 pinch cayenne pepper
1 pinch pink Himalayan salt
250 ml (9 fl oz/1 cup) hot rice
    milk
1 pinch ground cinnamon

Combine the carob powder, maca powder, cayenne pepper and salt in a latte glass. Top with the hot rice milk and stir well. Sprinkle with the ground cinnamon and serve immediately.

+ **NOTE** I love the earthy root flavour that maca gives to this drink. High in protein and good for overall wellbeing, maca grows in volcanic soils and the robust nature that survives a harsh climate is passed on to our bodies.

+ VEGETARIAN
+ VEGAN
+ GLUTEN-FREE
+ DAIRY-FREE
+ PALEO

PREP TIME:
5 minutes

COOKING TIME:
Nil

VELVET BEETROOT CACAO 'HUG-ME' LATTE

Getting into vegies is great. A plant-based diet is amazing and there are so many benefits of having more and more plant-based foods. This is a decadent yet very healthy drink. I call these 'hug-me' lattes as they really are like a hug in a mug.

SERVES 1

175 g (6 oz/about 1 large) beetroot
   (beet), scrubbed
1 tablespoon cacao powder
250 ml (9 fl oz/1 cup) hot almond
   milk
2 teaspoons raw honey,
   or use vegan sweetener

Push the beetroot through a juicer: you will need about 125 ml (4 fl oz/½ cup) juice. Transfer the juice to a mug and stir in the cacao powder. Stir the almond milk into the mug with the honey and serve immediately.

+ **NOTE** Cacao powder is high in magnesium, which helps to relax muscles, so you can drink this after dinner as a treat before going to bed.

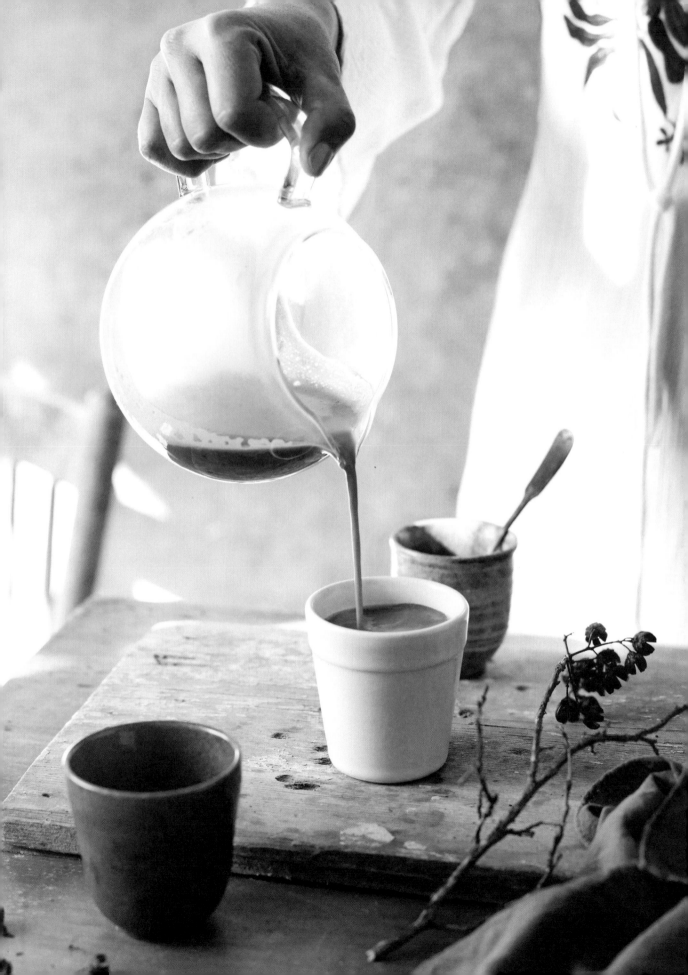

DIPS & SPREADS

PREP TIME:
10 minutes
COOKING TIME:
20 minutes

AYURVEDIC GINGER ARTICHOKE DIP

A creamy, satisfying and gut-healing dip.

MAKES 1 CUP

3 jerusalem artichokes, washed thoroughly
40 g (1½ oz/⅓ cup) chopped spring onions (scallions)
1 garlic clove
Juice of ½ lemon
1 tablespoon finely grated lemon zest
1 tablespoon olive oil
1 tablespoon finely grated ginger
1 teaspoon Digestive Spice (see page 175)
Superfood Crackers (see page 200), to serve

Put the artichokes in a saucepan of lightly salted cold water and bring to the boil over medium heat. Simmer for 15 minutes or until tender. Drain well.

Transfer the drained artichokes to a food processor, add the remaining ingredients with 1 tablespoon of water and process until smooth. Serve with crackers.

This dip is best eaten on the day of making.

+ **NOTE** Jerusalem artichoke is a great vegetable for your gut health as it has prebiotic fibre, which is great for growing good bacteria in your gut, keeping your immune system intact and strong.

+ VEGETARIAN
+ VEGAN
+ GLUTEN-FREE
+ DAIRY-FREE
+ PALEO

PREP TIME:
10 minutes

COOKING TIME:
Nil

CHIA OLIVE TAPENADE

This recipe is really easy to whip up. It's perfect to serve on a cheese platter and also makes a delicious marinade for chicken.

SERVES 3–4

150 g (5½ oz/1 cup) pitted black
    Kalamata olives
60 ml (2 fl oz/¼ cup) avocado oil
2 tablespoons capers in salt,
    rinsed well
60 g (2¼ oz/⅓ cup) chia seeds
1 garlic clove, chopped
1 tablespoon lemon juice
1 handful (about ½ cup) basil
    leaves

Put all of the ingredients in a blender with 60 ml (2 fl oz/¼ cup) of water and process to a paste. The tapenade is best eaten on the day of making.

+ **NOTE** Avocado oil: what an oil! Not only does it benefit heart health, it's also a source of good fats, a great balancer of moods and has beauty benefits for skin and hair.

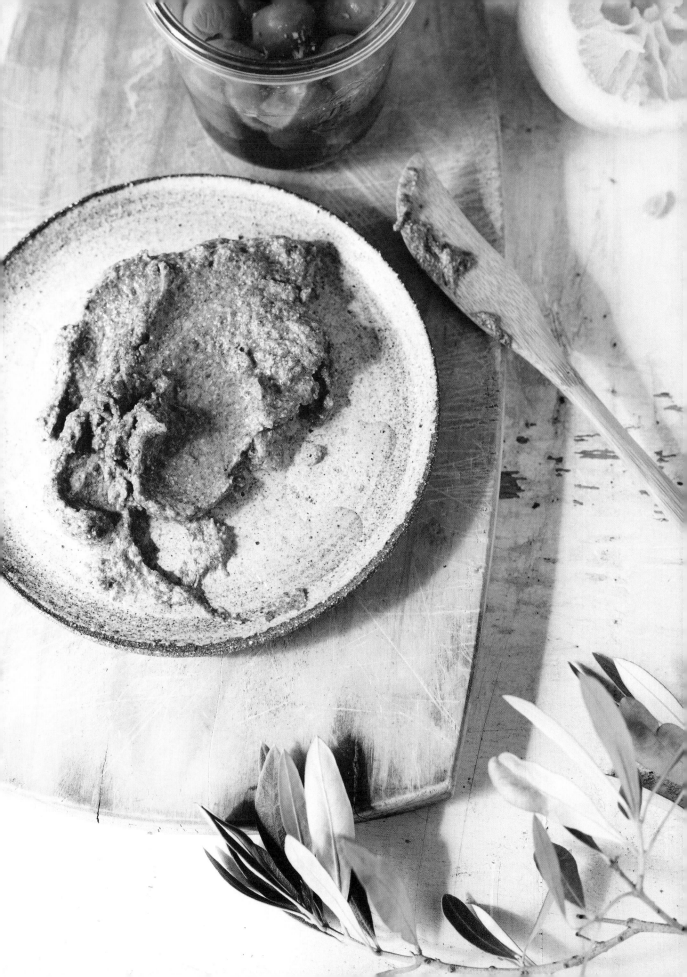

+ CREAMY MINT PESTO

+ ACTIVATED RAW KALE PESTO
(SEE PAGE 60 FOR RECIPE)

CREAMY MINT PESTO

This dip is so fresh and minty. I love the pairing of the tangy mint with the creamy cashews. Serve it as a dip, dressing or pasta sauce; use it on fish or with meat.

MAKES 1 CUP

135 g (4¾ oz/3 cups) baby spinach leaves
30 g (1 oz/1½ cups) mint leaves
10 g (⅜ oz/½ cup) flat-leaf (Italian) parsley leaves
80 g (2¾ oz/½ cup) raw cashews
80 g (2¾ oz/½ cup) pine nuts
50 g (1¾ oz/½ cup) grated parmesan cheese
60 ml (2 fl oz/¼ cup) olive oil, plus extra, to store
½ teaspoon salt
¼ teaspoon freshly ground black pepper
Juice of 1½ limes
60 ml (2 fl oz/¼ cup) kefir

Put all of the ingredients in a blender with 2 tablespoons of water and process until smooth. Transfer the pesto to a small airtight container, level the top, then pour a shallow layer of the extra olive oil over to prevent it from oxidising.

The pesto will keep for up to 3 days in an airtight container in the fridge.

+ **NOTE** I call spinach a superfood. Superfoods don't have to be hard to find or pronounce, so let's get some into our diets and use them as a foundation. I love using spinach in different dishes, smoothies and desserts. It is high in iron, great for bone health, muscles and eyesight and it's full of vitamins and minerals: get on it!

+ VEGETARIAN
+ VEGAN
+ GLUTEN-FREE
+ DAIRY-FREE
+ PALEO
+ RAW

PREP TIME:
*10 minutes,
plus drying and
overnight soaking*

COOKING TIME:
Nil

ACTIVATED RAW KALE PESTO

*This is one of our most popular dips; our
customers ask for the recipe all the time!
We get so many requests that I think including
it here will please many people.*

MAKES 1 CUP

155 g (5½ oz/1 cup) raw cashews
1 large kale leaf, finely chopped,
    stem removed (about 1 cup),
    or use cavolo nero
1 tablespoon apple cider vinegar
500 ml (17 fl oz/2 cups) warm
    water
1 tablespoon thinly sliced spring
    onions (scallions)
1 garlic clove
½ teaspoon pink Himalayan salt
1 pinch freshly ground black
    pepper
2 tablespoons lemon juice
125 ml (4 fl oz/½ cup) olive oil

Put the cashews in a bowl with 1 litre (35 fl oz/4 cups) of
water, cover and stand overnight or for at least 6 hours.

Preheat the oven to 40°C (105°F). Drain the cashews well,
then spread out on a baking tray and dry in the oven
for 1 hour.

Put the kale in a bowl, pour the vinegar and warm water
over and stand for 5 minutes. Drain the kale, then put it
in a blender with the remaining ingredients and the
dried cashews and blend until smooth.

––––––––

+ **NOTE** By soaking (activating) the cashews, you
    remove phytic acid and make more nutrients
    available for digestion. If you are time-poor you
    can purchase activated nuts or simply use the raw
    (unactivated) nuts.

PREP TIME:
*10 minutes,
plus 15 minutes
soaking*

COOKING TIME:
5 minutes

MUSHROOM, THYME & WALNUT PÂTÉ

*I love pâté and this is a great dip for entertaining
or you can use it as a spread on toast.*

SERVES 3–4

15 g (½ oz/½ cup) dried porcini
   mushrooms
15 g (½ oz/½ cup) dried shiitake
   mushrooms
250 ml (9 fl oz/1 cup) boiling
   water
60 g (2¼ oz/½ cup) raw walnuts
10 g (⅜ oz/⅓ cup) chopped
   flat-leaf (Italian) parsley
90 g (3¼ oz) unsalted butter,
   softened
20 g (¾ oz/⅓ cup) sliced spring
   onions (scallions)
1 teaspoon thyme leaves
1 teaspoon wholegrain or dijon
   mustard
3 teaspoons white chia seeds
¼ teaspoon salt
¼ teaspoon freshly ground black
   pepper
1 teaspoon olive oil

Soak the porcini and shiitake mushrooms together in the boiling water for 15 minutes.

Meanwhile, put the walnuts in a dry frying pan over medium heat and shake for 5 minutes or until toasted and golden.

Transfer the mushrooms and the soaking water to a blender, making sure you leave any gritty bits behind in the bottom of the bowl. Add the walnuts and all of the remaining ingredients, except the olive oil, and process until well combined; it does not have to be smooth. Transfer to a serving bowl and drizzle with the olive oil.

This pâté is best eaten on the day of making.

+ **NOTE** Shiitake mushrooms are great for immunity. Rich in vitamin B, they are great to use in many dishes. When using dried mushrooms, simply soak them in hot water, thinly slice and add to stir-fries, scrambled eggs, soups, curries, or use them along with the soaking water to make a mushroom sauce.

+ VEGETARIAN
+ VEGAN
+ GLUTEN-FREE
+ DAIRY-FREE
+ PALEO
+ RAW

PREP TIME:
10 minutes

COOKING TIME:
Nil

CHIA'ZY AVOCADO DIP

This dip is served in our café as a toast topper with cherry tomatoes and chopped coriander (cilantro) and is a top seller. People go crazy for it: it's simple, yet the ingredients work well together, delivering a tasty dish for breakfast or lunch. Once we'd published this recipe, it was an instant winner, so we've repeated it here.

MAKES 1 CUP

2 ripe avocados
2 tablespoons savoury yeast
    flakes
Juice of ½ lemon
1 handful (about ½ cup) basil
    leaves
1 tablespoon chia seeds
¼ teaspoon cayenne pepper
¼ teaspoon Celtic sea salt
2 tablespoons olive oil
1 tablespoon water

Put all of the ingredients into a blender and blend until smooth.

This dip is best eaten on the day of making.

+ **NOTE** Savoury yeast flakes are a rich source of B vitamins. They add a cheesy flavour to a variety of dishes such as soups, dips, baked vegies and pasta.

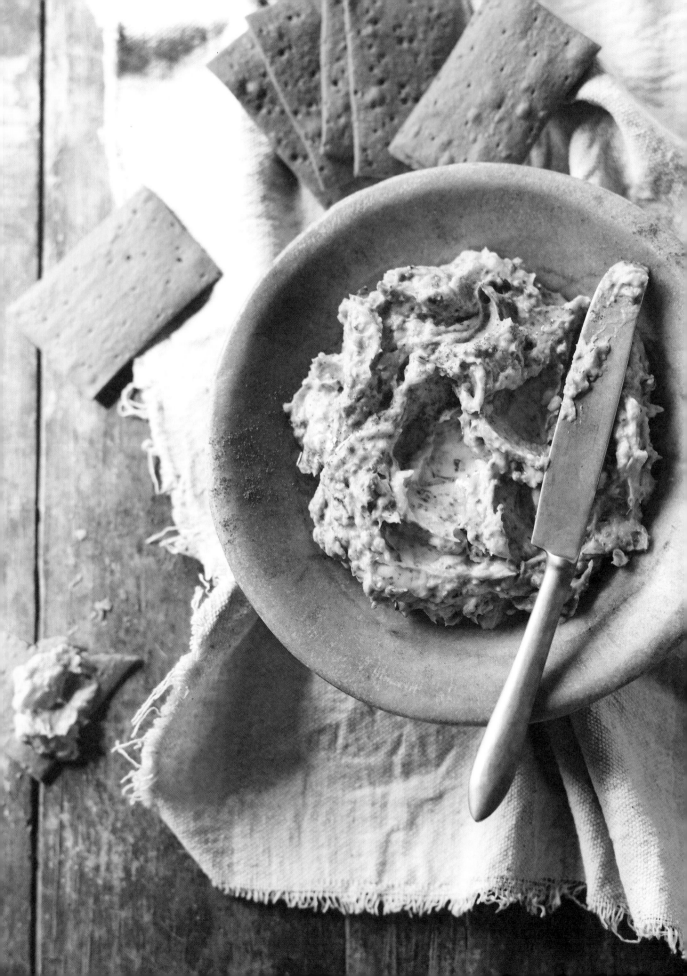

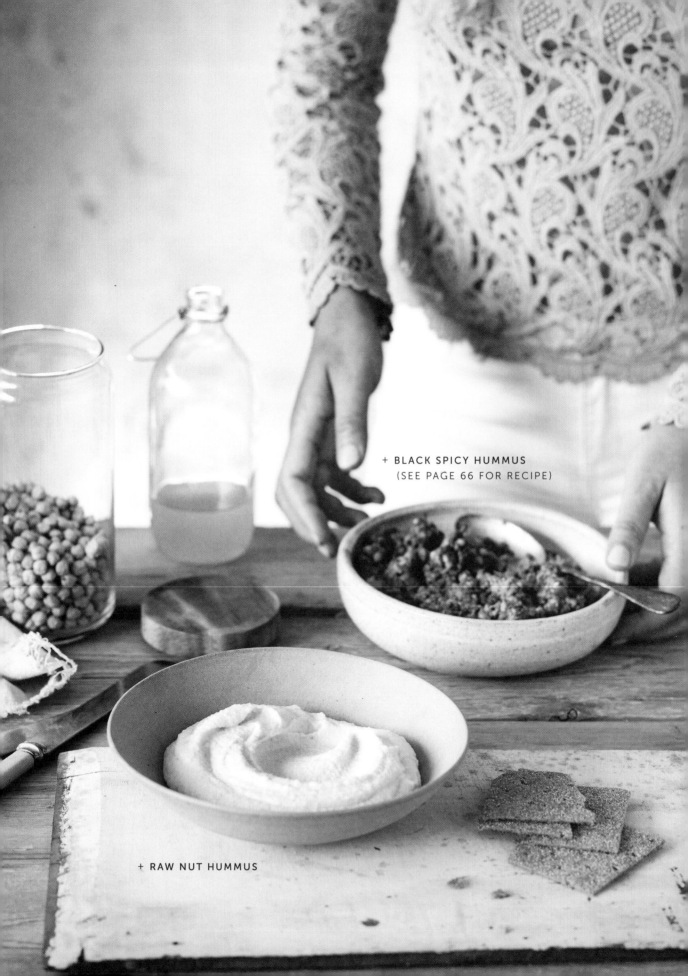

+ BLACK SPICY HUMMUS
(SEE PAGE 66 FOR RECIPE)

+ RAW NUT HUMMUS

+ VEGETARIAN
+ VEGAN
+ GLUTEN-FREE
+ DAIRY-FREE
+ PALEO
+ RAW

PREP TIME:
10 minutes, plus overnight soaking

COOKING TIME:
Nil

RAW NUT HUMMUS

A top seller in our stores, this vegan hummus is creamy and nutty.

MAKES 1 CUP

310 g (11 oz/2 cups) raw cashews
230 g (8¼ oz) almond meal
125 ml (4 fl oz/½ cup) olive oil
2 tablespoons tahini
2 tablespoons lemon juice
2 garlic cloves
2 teaspoons ground cumin
1 teaspoon salt
1 pinch freshly ground black
   pepper

Put the cashews and 1 litre (35 fl oz/4 cups) of water in a bowl and soak overnight.

The following day, drain the cashews, then put them in a blender with all of the remaining ingredients and pulse until coarsely chopped. Add 185 ml (6 fl oz/¾ cup) of water and process until smooth. Check the seasoning and add more salt if desired.

The hummus will keep for up to 5 days in an airtight container in the fridge.

+ **NOTE** Don't avoid eating cashews because they are fatty! They contain a good type of fat — mostly unsaturated — which can help lower cholesterol levels and improve heart health.

+ VEGETARIAN
+ VEGAN
+ GLUTEN-FREE
+ DAIRY-FREE
+ PALEO

PREP TIME:
10 minutes

COOKING TIME:
1 hour 35 minutes

BLACK SPICY HUMMUS

This is not stereotypical hummus: it has a crunchy texture and is great on top of a salad as extra plant protein. I often whip this up for friends and the question I'm always asked is, 'What makes it black?' Simple, it's the tahini made from black sesame seeds. Black foods are nutrient rich: in general, the darker the food, the more nutrients are in it. I love using black tahini in not only savoury dishes but also in sweets, such as my Black Tahini Smoothie (see page 41).

MAKES 2 CUPS

200 g (7 oz/1 cup) dried chickpeas, soaked overnight in cold water
2 tablespoons apple cider vinegar
2 tablespoons linseed (flaxseed) oil
1 tablespoon linseeds (flaxseeds)
65 g (2½ oz/¼ cup) black tahini
1 teaspoon pink Himalayan salt
¼ teaspoon freshly ground black pepper
¼ teaspoon cayenne pepper
2 tablespoons water
Olive oil, to drizzle

Drain the soaked chickpeas, then put them in a saucepan and cover with plenty of lightly salted cold water. Bring to the boil over high heat, then reduce the heat to low and simmer for 1½ hours or until tender. Drain well.

Transfer the chickpeas and all of the remaining ingredients to a blender and blend until combined but still a little chunky. Adjust the seasoning if desired.

Drizzle with olive oil. The hummus will keep for up to 5 days in an airtight container in the fridge.

+ **NOTE** Chickpeas are a vegetarian-friendly protein: they give an amazing creamy texture to any dish. If you're in a hurry, you can use 400 g (14 oz/2 cups) of tinned chickpeas instead of soaking and cooking.

BAOBAB & ORANGE CHIA JAM

Use this jam as a spread, in smoothies and with pancakes or as a topping over chocolate ice cream. Black chia seeds provide a lovely contrast with the orange colour.

MAKES ABOUT 1½ CUPS

3 oranges
1 lemon
1 cinnamon stick
3 cloves
115 g (4 oz/⅓ cup) honey
2 tablespoons black chia seeds
3 tablespoons baobab powder

Peel 2 of the oranges and the lemon, then coarsely chop the flesh. Put the flesh in a blender and blitz until mushy, then transfer to a saucepan. Slice the remaining orange into thin wedges, then add to the pan with the cinnamon stick, cloves, honey and 60 ml (2 fl oz/¼ cup) of water. Bring to the boil, reduce the heat to low and cook for 15 minutes.

Remove from the heat, discarding the cinnamon stick and cloves. Stir in the chia seeds, then allow to cool in the saucepan. Stir in the baobab powder, then spoon the jam into an airtight container and refrigerate for up to 5 days.

+ **NOTE** Baobab powder gives a vitamin C boost, which contributes to collagen formation: I call it natural Botox! Baobab also helps with the absorption of iron.

+ VEGETARIAN
+ VEGAN
+ GLUTEN-FREE
+ DAIRY-FREE
+ PALEO
+ RAW

PREP TIME:
5 minutes

COOKING TIME:
Nil

RAW RASPBERRY CHIA JAM

This jam is an About Life classic and one of my favourite quick and easy recipes. It's easy to make and you can create different flavours by simply swapping the fruit: try blueberries, strawberries or blackberries, or any combination. Pair it with bit of almond butter or yoghurt for slow-releasing sugars. I like it quite tart, but if you have a sweet tooth you can add more dates.

MAKES 1½ CUPS

375 g (13 oz/3 cups) frozen
    raspberries, slightly defrosted
4 whole dates, pitted
3 tablespoons white chia seeds
¼ teaspoon vanilla bean paste

Combine all of the ingredients in a blender, add 2 tablespoons of water and blend until smooth.

The jam will keep for 7–10 days in an airtight container in the fridge.

+ **NOTE** Raspberries are high in antioxidants and low in fructose, so they will not cause blood sugar levels to spike.

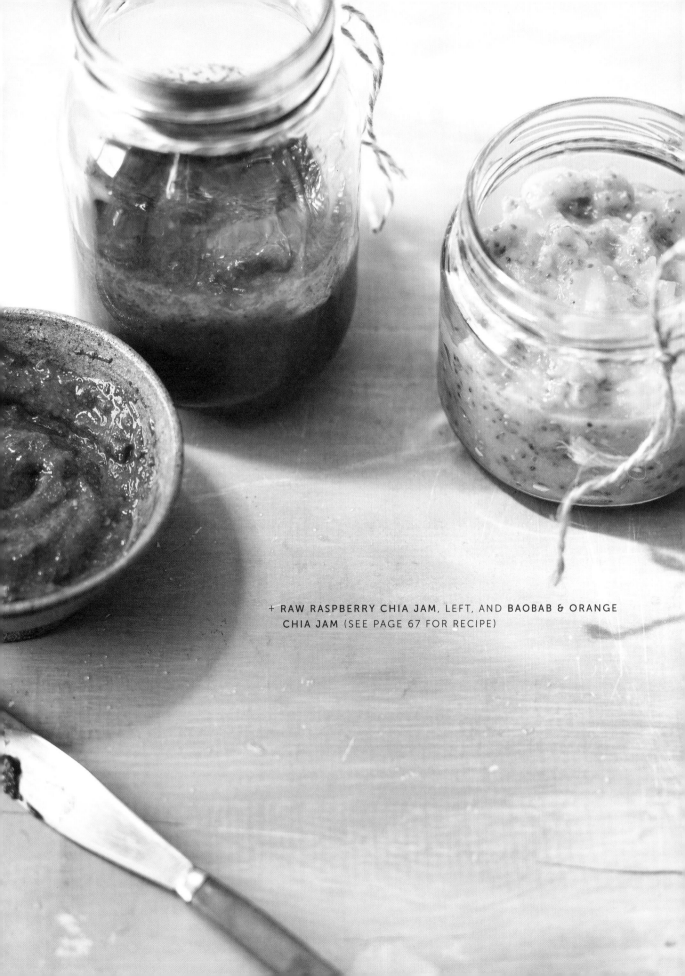

+ RAW RASPBERRY CHIA JAM, LEFT, AND BAOBAB & ORANGE CHIA JAM (SEE PAGE 67 FOR RECIPE)

SALADS

+ VEGETARIAN
+ GLUTEN-FREE
+ DAIRY-FREE

PREP TIME:
*30 minutes, plus
10 minutes standing*

COOKING TIME:
5 minutes

CRUNCHY CHIA TOFU WITH BROWN RICE NOODLES

This is a salad to serve on any meatless Monday.

SERVES 4

200 g (7 oz) dried brown rice
    noodles
125 ml (4 fl oz/½ cup) coconut oil
1 tablespoon sesame oil
350 g (12 oz) block firm tofu,
    cut into small cubes
2 tablespoons tamari (gluten-free
    soy sauce)
3 tablespoons black chia seeds
50 g (1¾ oz/⅓ cup) sesame seeds,
    toasted
2 carrots, grated
2 Lebanese (short) cucumbers,
    halved lengthways, seeded
    and sliced
2 red capsicums (peppers), seeded
    and finely chopped
60 g (2¼ oz/½ cup) thinly sliced
    spring onions (scallions)
3 tablespoons chopped coriander
    (cilantro) leaves
2 tablespoons chopped mint
1 quantity Umeboshi Dressing
    (see page 86)
3 sheets nori
80 g (2¾ oz/½ cup) raw cashews,
    coarsely chopped

Put the brown rice noodles in a bowl and cover with just-boiled water. Stand for 10 minutes or until tender. Drain and set aside.

Heat the coconut oil and sesame oil in a frying pan over medium heat. Cook the tofu cubes, turning often for about 4 minutes or until golden. Add the tamari and cook for another minute, then remove from the heat. Remove the tofu from the oil using tongs and drain on paper towel. Combine the chia seeds and sesame seeds in a large bowl. Add the hot tofu and toss to coat well.

Put the vegetables, herbs, tofu and drained noodles in a large bowl. Season with salt and freshly ground black pepper and toss to combine. Pour the umeboshi dressing over the noodle salad, toss to combine well, then transfer to a serving dish. Using a pair of scissors, chop the nori sheets into narrow strips and scatter over the top, sprinkle with the chopped cashews and serve.

+ **NOTE** Brown rice noodles are made from whole brown rice. They're great complex carbohydrates that release more slowly, giving lasting energy. When choosing noodles and pasta, always go for brown wholegrains.

PREP TIME:
15 minutes

COOKING TIME:
10 minutes

DECONSTRUCTED NOURISHING SUSHI BOWL

This sushi bowl is a lunch or dinner salad, with fibre, carbohydrates, protein and good fats.

SERVES 2

1 tablespoon olive oil
1 small red (Spanish) onion, finely chopped
1 garlic clove, thinly sliced
1 tablespoon finely chopped fresh ginger
370 g (13 oz/2 cups) cooked brown rice
70 g (2½ oz) snow peas (mangetout), trimmed
80 g (2¾ oz) green beans, trimmed and halved
2 tablespoons tamari (gluten-free soy sauce)
1 large kale leaf, thinly sliced, stalk removed (about 1 cup)
1 tablespoon lemon juice
1 small carrot, sliced into ribbons
2 nori sheets, torn into pieces
185 g (6½ oz) tinned tuna in oil, drained
2 tablespoons black chia seeds
1 avocado
2 tablespoons Miso Coriander Dressing (see page 154)
2 tablespoons sesame seeds
Lemon wedges and Pickled Kimchi (see page 171), to serve

Heat the olive oil in a large frying pan over medium heat. Add the onion and cook for 5–6 minutes until soft. Add the garlic, ginger and cooked brown rice and stir until heated through. Stir in the snow peas, beans and tamari, followed by the kale. Drizzle the lemon juice over, then remove from the heat and divide between two bowls.

Top each bowl with half each of the carrot, torn nori and tuna, keeping each ingredient separate. Halve the avocado lengthways and discard the skin and stone. Spread the chia seeds on a plate, dip one side of each avocado half into the seeds, then add to the bowl. We eat with our eyes so take your time arranging the toppings! Add a drizzle of raw miso dressing over each salad bowl and top with the sesame seeds. Serve with wedges of lemon and a little kimchi or other fermented vegetables.

+ **NOTE** For 370 g (13 oz/2 cups) of brown rice, put 310 ml (10¾ fl oz/1¼ cups) of water in a saucepan, add salt and bring to the boil. Add 110 g (3¾ oz/½ cup) uncooked brown rice, reduce heat to low and cook for 30 minutes or until water is absorbed and rice is tender. Fluff with a fork.

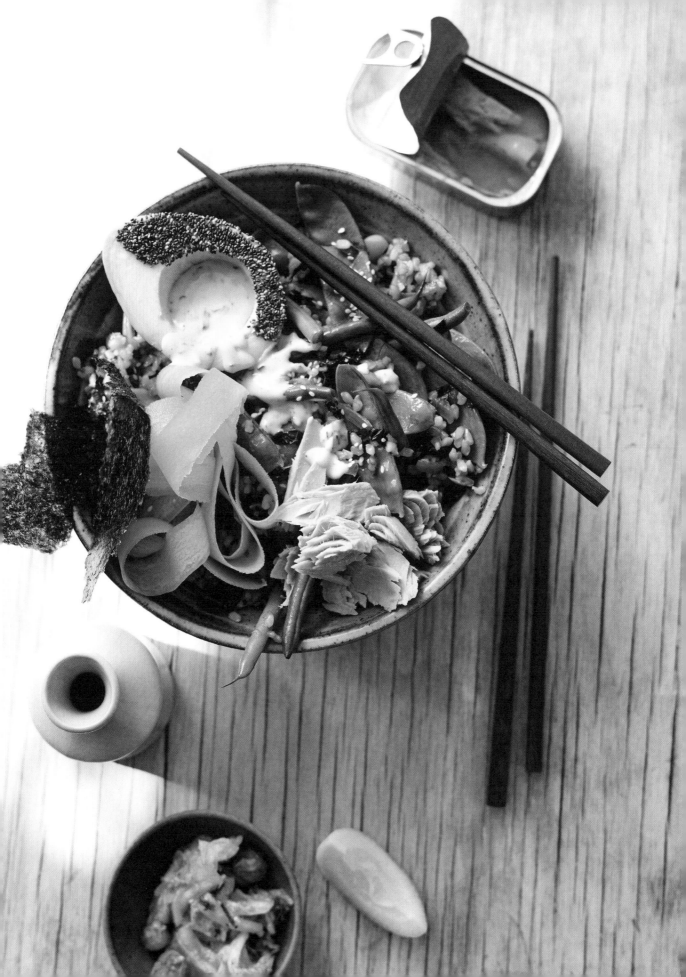

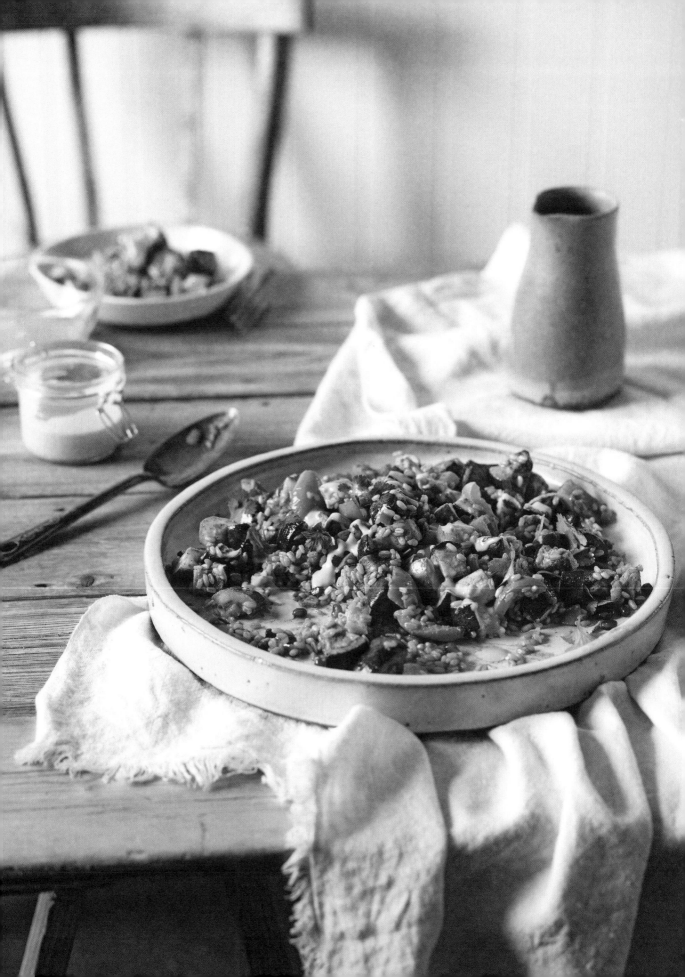

+ VEGETARIAN
+ VEGAN
+ DAIRY-FREE

PREP TIME:
20 minutes, plus overnight soaking and 1 hour cooling

COOKING TIME:
1 hour 20 minutes

JEWELLED FREEKEH SALAD

This colourful plate of goodness and flavour is a fantastic accompaniment to any protein dish.

SERVES 4

200 g (7 oz/1 cup) whole wheat freekeh
2 zucchini (courgettes), cut into 2 cm (¾ inch) pieces
1 large eggplant (aubergine), cut into 2 cm (¾ inch) pieces
2 red capsicums (peppers), seeds and membranes removed, cut into 2 cm (¾ inch) pieces
1 red (Spanish) onion, finely chopped
2 teaspoons sweet paprika
1 teaspoon ground cumin
1 teaspoon ground cinnamon
2 teaspoons ground turmeric
1 teaspoon ground coriander
¼ teaspoon salt
2 tablespoons olive oil
Seeds of ½ pomegranate (see note on page 81)
15 g (½ oz/½ cup) coriander (cilantro) leaves
Hulled tahini, to drizzle

DRESSING
Zest and juice of ½ orange
2 tablespoons lemon juice
60 ml (2 fl oz/¼ cup) olive oil

Soak the freekeh overnight in cold water. The following day, drain the freekeh. Put it in a saucepan with 750 ml (26 fl oz/3 cups) of lightly salted water and bring to the boil over high heat. Reduce the heat to low, cover and cook for 35–40 minutes until tender. Remove from the heat and stand, covered, until cool.

Preheat the oven to 180°C (350°F).

Put all of the vegetables into a large mixing bowl, add the spices and olive oil and mix well. Spread the vegetables on a large baking tray and roast for 30 minutes or until golden and slightly soft.

Meanwhile, to make the dressing, mix all of the ingredients in a small bowl and whisk to combine well.

To serve, put the freekeh and roasted vegetables in a large salad bowl. Add the dressing and toss to coat. Scatter with the pomegranate seeds, coriander leaves and drizzle with hulled tahini.

+ **NOTE** Freekeh is wholegrain young green wheat full of health benefits: it is high in protein, dietary fibre, vitamins and minerals – in particular, calcium, potassium, iron and zinc.

+ VEGETARIAN
+ VEGAN
+ GLUTEN-FREE
+ DAIRY-FREE
+ PALEO
+ RAW

PREP TIME:
*15 minutes,
plus 15 minutes
standing*

COOKING TIME:
Nil

SIGNATURE KALE & CARROT SALAD

*So simple to make and it's a best seller.
Serve with fish or chicken, and add avocado.*

SERVES 4

4 carrots, shredded
2 bunches kale, thinly sliced,
    stalks removed, or use
    cavolo nero
60 ml (2 fl oz/¼ cup) sesame oil
80 ml (2½ fl oz/⅓ cup) apple cider
    vinegar
75 g (2¾ oz/½ cup) sesame seeds

DRESSING
135 g (4¾ oz/½ cup) tahini
Juice of 1 lemon
½ teaspoon salt
80 ml (2½ fl oz/⅓ cup) olive oil

Put the carrot, kale, sesame oil and vinegar in a large bowl and massage with your hands for 3 minutes. Set aside for 10–15 minutes until softened.

Meanwhile, to make the dressing, combine all of the ingredients in a bowl, add 125 ml (4 fl oz/½ cup) of water and stir until well combined.

To serve, transfer the kale and carrot mixture (including any liquid) to a serving bowl, drizzle with half the dressing and scatter with the sesame seeds. Serve the remaining dressing on the side. Leftover dressing will keep in an airtight container in the fridge for up to 1 week.

+ **NOTE** Massaging kale begins the digestion process by starting to break the leaves down. Preparing your food this way means you will absorb more nutrients.

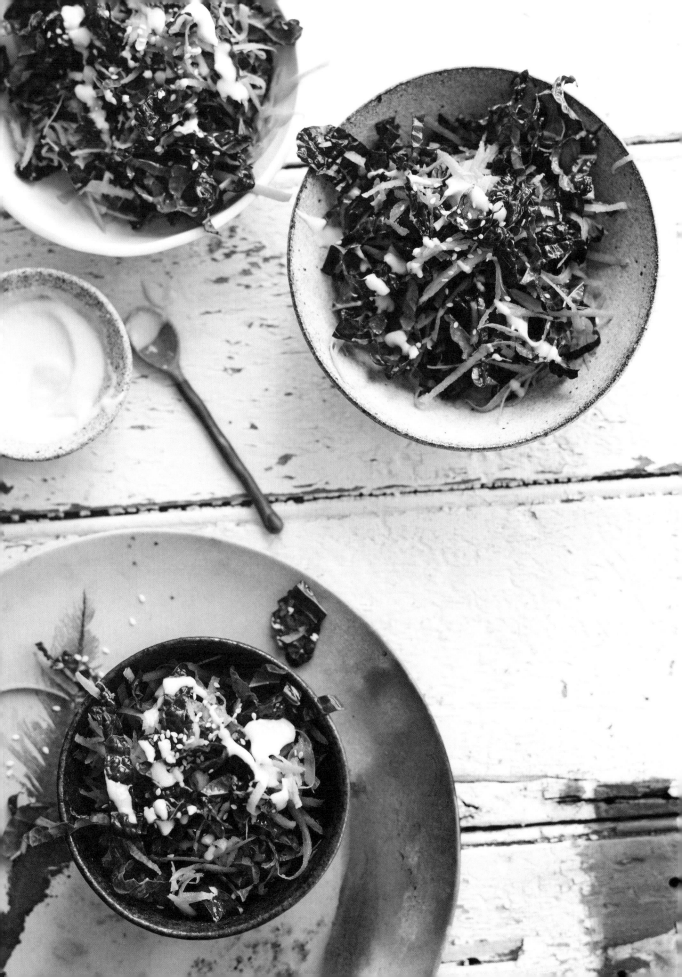

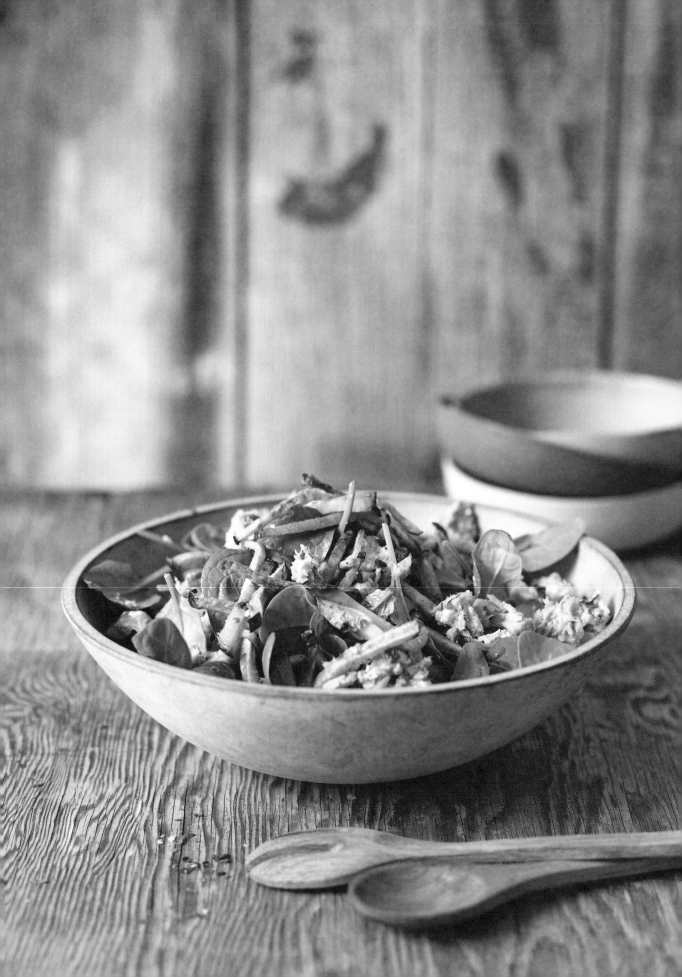

ENERGISING COCONUT & SWEET POTATO SALAD

A surprisingly delicious dance of ingredients.

SERVES 4 AS A MAIN COURSE

60 ml (2 fl oz/¼ cup) melted
    coconut oil
2 large (about 900 g/2 lb) sweet
    potatoes (any colour)
90 g (3¼ oz/⅓ cup) tahini
380 g (13½ oz) tinned tuna in oil,
    drained
180 g (6¼ oz) feta cheese,
    crumbled
Juice of 1 lemon
180 g (6¼ oz/4 cups) baby spinach
    leaves
1 pinch each salt and freshly
    ground black pepper
1 pinch dried chilli flakes

Preheat the oven to 200°C (400°F). Lightly grease a large baking tray with the coconut oil. Using a mandolin or large sharp knife, thinly slice the sweet potato into rounds about 3 mm (⅛ inch) thick. Cut the rounds into straws about the same width.

Combine the sweet potato straws with the remaining coconut oil and spread on the baking tray and season with salt and pepper. Bake for 30–40 minutes until golden brown.

In a large bowl combine the tahini, tuna, feta and lemon juice, then toss through the sweet potato chips. Add the spinach and toss well. Sprinkle with chilli to serve.

+ **NOTE** You can find various types of sweet potato: there are purple, red, pale yellow or white varieties as well as the orange ones. Sweet potatoes are rich in antioxidants: the more intense the colour of the vegetable, the more antioxidants it contains, so choose colourful sweet potatoes for consumption, especially the purple and red ones.

+ GLUTEN-FREE
+ DAIRY-FREE
+ PALEO

PREP TIME:
30 minutes

COOKING TIME:
25 minutes

ALMOND BUTTER KELP NOODLE SALAD

A beautiful peanut-free satay sauce–inspired salad.

SERVES 4

120 g (4¼ oz/¾ cup) raw almond
    kernels
30 g (1 oz/¾ cup) coconut chips
800 g (1 lb 12 oz) fresh kelp
    noodles
125 ml (4 fl oz/½ cup) tinned
    coconut milk
80 ml (2½ fl oz/⅓ cup) lime juice
2 teaspoons spirulina powder
90 g (3¼ oz/⅓ cup) almond butter
60 ml (2 fl oz/¼ cup) tamari
    (gluten-free soy sauce)
150 g (5½ oz) snow peas
    (mangetout), trimmed
200 g (7 oz) broccoli, cut into
    small florets
2 red capsicums (peppers), seeds
    and membranes removed,
    thinly sliced
1 tablespoon coconut oil
650 g (1 lb 7 oz) skinless chicken
    thigh fillets, cut into strips
2 tablespoons coriander (cilantro)
    leaves
Lime wedges and thinly sliced
    fresh red chilli, to serve

Preheat the oven to 180°C (350°F). Spread the almonds and coconut chips on separate baking trays and bake for 10 minutes or until just golden. Remove from the oven, coarsely chop the almonds and set aside.

Meanwhile, rinse the kelp noodles under cold running water, then drain well.

Combine the coconut milk, lime juice, spirulina powder, almond butter and tamari in a large bowl. Add the vegetables and the drained noodles, season with salt and freshly ground black pepper and toss to combine well. Transfer to a serving platter.

Heat a large, shallow frying pan over medium heat. When hot, add the coconut oil, then the chicken strips and cook for 6–8 minutes on each side until golden. Drain on paper towel.

To serve, place the warm chicken on top of the noodle salad. Scatter with the toasted almonds and coconut chips, then the coriander leaves. Serve with lime wedges and fresh chilli.

+ NOTE Almond butter is a delicious way to add essential proteins, vitamins and minerals to your diet. Use it in salad dressings, smoothies, or even with fruit and yoghurt to make ice cream.

PREP TIME:
*10 minutes, plus
20 minutes standing
and cooling*

COOKING TIME:
30 minutes

BLACK RICE WITH POMEGRANATE, EDAMAME, MINT & FETA

*Colourful, fresh and tasty, black rice offers
a dramatic look. A splash of red from the
pomegranate and the bright green edamame
make a picturesque presentation on the plate.*

SERVES 4

400 g (14 oz/2 cups) black rice
2 pomegranates, seeds removed
   (see note)
200 g (7 oz/2 cups) shelled
   edamame
260 g (9¼ oz) feta cheese,
   crumbled
2 large handfuls mint leaves
½ teaspoon salt

DRESSING
80 ml (2½ fl oz/⅓ cup) apple cider
   vinegar
80 ml (2½ fl oz/⅓ cup) extra
   virgin olive oil

Put the black rice in a saucepan with 1 litre
(35 fl oz/4 cups) of water and bring to the boil over
high heat. Reduce the heat to low and simmer for
20–30 minutes until the rice is soft. Remove from the
heat, cover and stand for 10 minutes. Transfer the rice
to a bowl and set aside to cool.

To make the dressing, whisk together the vinegar
and olive oil.

When the rice is cool, add the pomegranate seeds,
edamame, feta, mint and salt. Pour the dressing over,
stir to combine well and serve.

+ **NOTE** I find the best way to remove the seeds from
   a pomegranate is to use a small sharp knife to score
   four lines from the top of the pomegranate to the
   bottom. Submerge the pomegranate in a bowl of cold
   water, then pull the quarters apart, releasing the seeds
   with your hands. The pith will float to the top and
   the seeds will sink.

SMOKED TROUT WITH GOLDEN HORSERADISH LABNEH & BUSH GREENS

*I love using bush foods and spices in recipes.
In this recipe I have used chickweed, which brings
an earthy, slightly grassy taste that reminds me of
playing as a child: it's lovely that food can spark
amazing memories.*

SERVES 4

4 medium beetroot (beets),
   scrubbed
60 ml (2 fl oz/¼ cup) extra virgin
   olive oil
2 tablespoons balsamic vinegar
¼ teaspoon each salt and freshly
   ground black pepper
200 g (7 oz/3 cups) chickweed
450 g (1 lb) hot-smoked trout,
   skin and bones discarded
125 g (4½ fl oz/½ cup) Golden
   Labneh (see page 136)
3 tablespoons freshly grated
   horseradish
30 g (1 oz/½ cup) dill sprigs
   (optional)

Preheat the oven to 200°C (400°F).

Wrap each beetroot in foil and bake for 45 minutes or until a skewer inserts easily. Remove from the oven and, when cool enough to handle, peel and cut the beets into thin wedges.

Meanwhile, whisk the olive oil, balsamic vinegar, salt and pepper together to make the dressing.

Put the beetroot slices, chickweed and dressing in a mixing bowl and toss to coat. Place on a large salad plate and flake the smoked trout over the top.

Combine the Golden Labneh and horseradish in a small bowl and whisk them together with a fork. Dollop on top of the salad, then scatter the dill sprigs over (if using) and serve.

+ **NOTE** Other bush greens include chicory and Australian native warrigal greens. If you can't find any of these, you can use rocket (arugula) and baby spinach leaves.

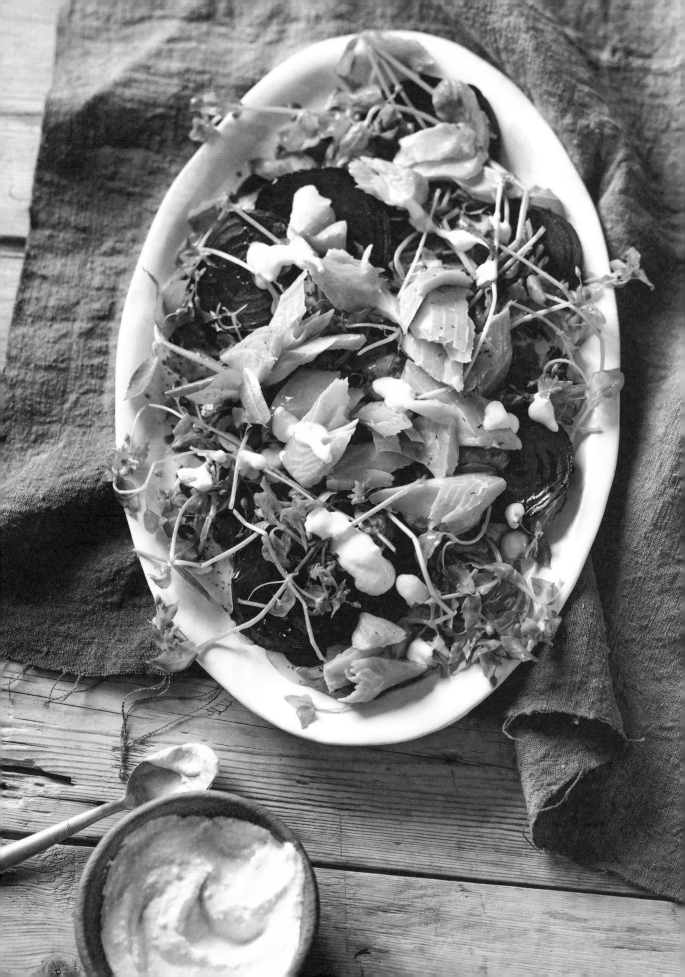

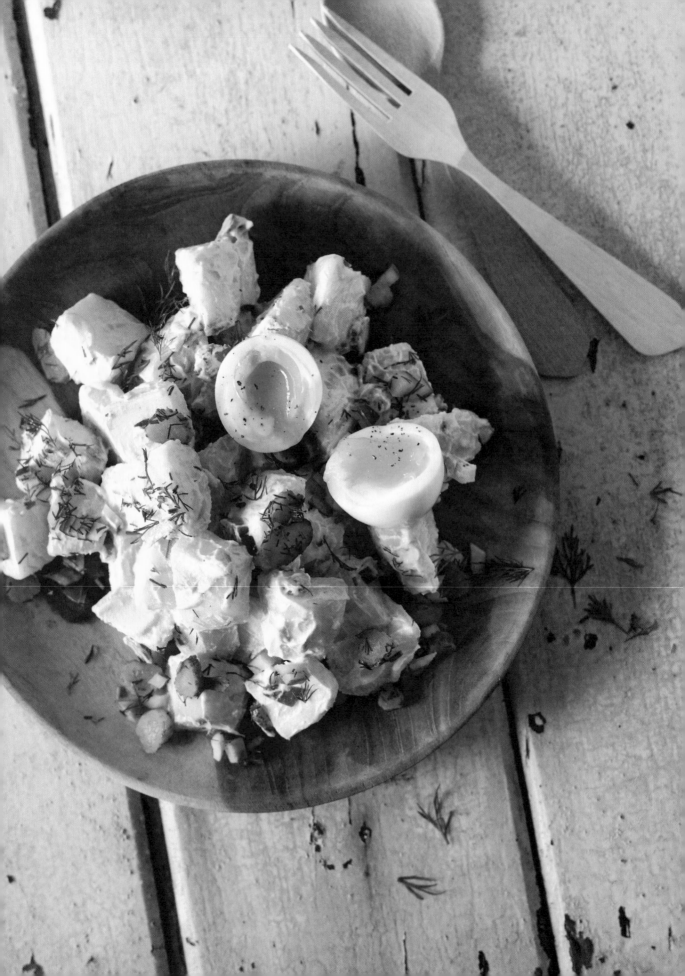

PREP TIME:
15 minutes, plus
30 minutes cooling

COOKING TIME:
20 minutes

THE BEST TURMERIC YOGHURT & TAHINI POTATO SALAD

The best creamy potato salad (thanks to the tahini and yoghurt) without the guilt! Adding gherkins gives it a little zest. Delicious served with Crispy Coconut Chicken (see page 126) or Lemon & Thyme Macadamia Crusted Fish (see page 152).

SERVES 2 AS A MAIN OR 4 AS A SIDE

450 g (1 lb/about 5 small) potatoes (sebago, dutch cream or desiree), peeled and cut into 2–3 cm (¾–1¼ inch) pieces
2 eggs
½ red (Spanish) onion, finely chopped
2 tablespoons thinly sliced cornichons (small pickles), 80 ml (2½ oz/⅓ cup) pickling liquid reserved
1 tablespoon chopped dill
½ teaspoon salt
130 g (4½ oz/½ cup) buffalo yoghurt, or Greek-style yoghurt
90 g (3¼ oz/⅓ cup) tahini
2 tablespoons olive oil
2 tablespoons dijon mustard
1 teaspoon ground turmeric

Put the potatoes in a saucepan, cover with lightly salted cold water and bring to the boil. Simmer over medium heat for 15 minutes or until tender but not falling apart. Drain and set aside to cool.

Meanwhile, soft-boil the eggs by putting them in a saucepan of cold water. Bring to the boil and cook over high heat for 3 minutes. Transfer the eggs to a bowl of cold water and rest for 1 minute, then drain and peel off shells.

Transfer the cooled potatoes to a large bowl. Add the onion, gherkin, dill and salt.

Whisk together the yoghurt, tahini, olive oil, reserved pickling liquid, mustard and turmeric, then pour over the potatoes and toss gently to coat. Adjust the seasoning if necessary.

Put the salad in a serving bowl and top with the soft-boiled eggs, gently pulled in half.

+ VEGETARIAN
+ VEGAN
+ GLUTEN-FREE
+ DAIRY-FREE

PREP TIME:
15 minutes
COOKING TIME:
20 minutes

UMEBOSHI BLACK BEAN SPAGHETTI SALAD WITH SESAME TOASTED BROCCOLI

The black bean spaghetti gives a great colour contrast to the green vegies. It's a perfect match.

SERVES 4

200 g (7 oz) broccoli, cut into
    small florets
1 tablespoon sesame oil
1 tablespoon sesame seeds
200 g (7 oz) black bean spaghetti
    (or brown rice noodles)
150 g (5½ oz) snow peas
    (mangetout), trimmed and
    halved lengthways
250 g (9 oz) green beans, trimmed
    and cut in half

UMEBOSHI DRESSING
60 ml (2 fl oz/¼ cup) sesame oil
1½ tablespoons mirin (rice wine)
2 tablespoons umeboshi
    (fermented Japanese
    plum) paste
¼ cup finely grated fresh ginger
75 g (2¾ oz/½ cup) sesame seeds
1 tablespoon tamari (gluten-free
    soy sauce)

Preheat the oven to 180°C (350°F).

Spread the broccoli on a baking tray, add the sesame oil and sesame seeds and toss to combine. Bake for 20 minutes or until lightly roasted but still crunchy.

Meanwhile, bring 2 litres (70 fl oz/8 cups) of water to the boil in a large saucepan over high heat. Add the spaghetti and cook for 6–8 minutes until tender. Add the snow peas and green beans for the last minute of cooking to blanch. Drain and rinse under cold water to stop the cooking process.

To make the dressing, whisk all the ingredients together in a small bowl with 60 ml (2 fl oz/¼ cup) of water.

Transfer the spaghetti, snow peas and green beans to a serving bowl. Pour in the dressing and toss until well coated. Top with the crunchy broccoli florets and serve.

+ **NOTE** Umeboshi paste is made from fermented plums: it has a salty flavour yet still tastes like a plum. It is absolutely delicious and has antiviral properties. Try it as a pick-me-up when you're run down.

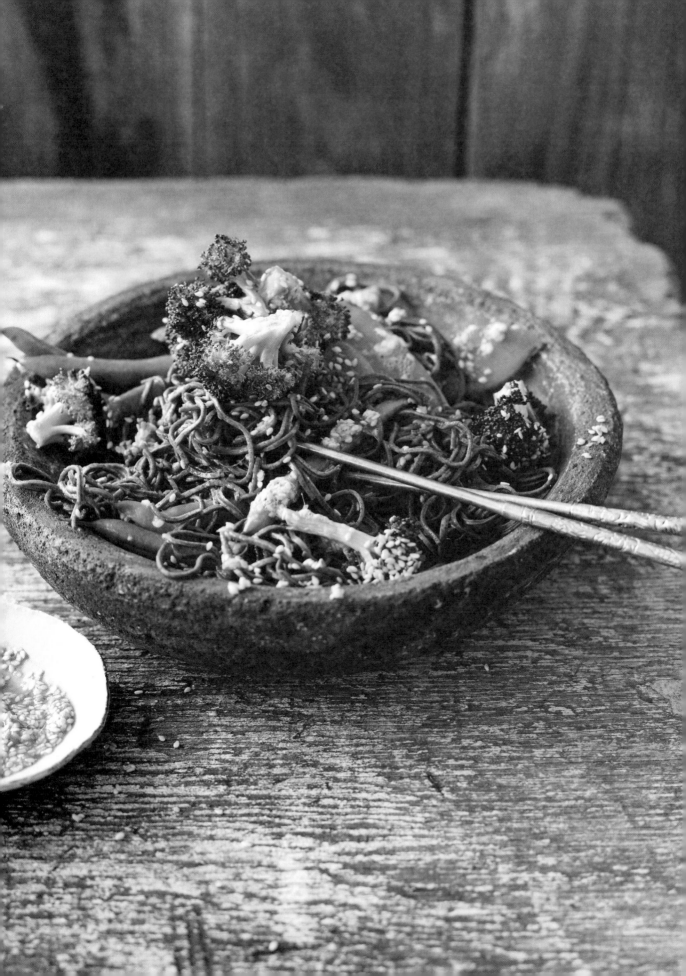

WARM BEETROOT, AVOCADO & GOAT'S FETA SALAD

This classic salad uses not just the beetroot, but the leaves as well.

SERVES 4

1 bunch (about 500 g/1 lb 2 oz) whole beetroot (beets)
60 ml (2 fl oz/¼ cup) olive oil
1 garlic clove, chopped
1 tablespoon lemon juice
¼ teaspoon salt
1 pinch freshly ground black pepper
180 g (6¼ oz/4 cups) baby spinach leaves
1 avocado, halved lengthways, skin and stone discarded, diced
3 spring onions (scallions), thinly sliced
130 g (4½ oz) goat's feta cheese, crumbled
75 g (2¾ oz/½ cup) pepitas (pumpkin seeds)

DRESSING
2 tablespoons sunflower seed butter (or use almond butter)
Juice of ½ lemon
1 tablespoon raw honey
60 ml (2 fl oz/¼ cup) apple cider vinegar
60 ml (2 fl oz/¼ cup) extra virgin olive oil

Preheat the oven to 180°C (350°F). Trim the leafy tops off the beetroot, rinse well and set aside. Scrub the beetroot and spread on a baking tray. Drizzle with 1 tablespoon of the olive oil, ensuring each beet is well coated. Cover the tray with foil and bake for 1½ hours or until a skewer goes in easily. The cooking time will vary depending on how large the beets are so check them occasionally.

Meanwhile, to make the dressing, whisk all of the ingredients together in a small bowl, season with salt and freshly ground black pepper and set aside.

When the beetroots are ready, remove them from the oven, uncover and allow to cool for 5 minutes. Remove the skin, then dice and put into a large bowl.

Heat the remaining olive oil in a large frying pan over medium heat. Add the garlic and reserved beetroot leaves and toss for 2 minutes or until the leaves are slightly wilted. Remove from the heat, then add the lemon juice, salt and pepper and toss to combine.

Add the wilted beetroot leaves, spinach leaves, avocado and spring onion to the beetroot and pour the dressing over. Toss the salad lightly: the heat from the beets and wilted leaves will break down the spinach slightly. Transfer to a shallow serving bowl, scatter with the crumbled feta and the pepitas and serve.

CELERY SALAD WITH BLUE CHEESE & APPLE

I really like to use the pale outer leaves of the cauliflower along with the celery leaves in this salad.

SERVES 4

1 cauliflower, about 800 g–1 kg
   (1 lb 12 oz–2 lb 4 oz)
2 tablespoons Digestive Spice
   (see page 175)
2 teaspoons melted coconut oil
3 granny smith apples, cored
   and thinly sliced
4–6 celery stalks, grated
3 cups celery leaves
250 g (9 oz) Roquefort cheese,
   crumbled

Preheat the oven to 200°C (400°F).

Cut the cauliflower into small florets, reserving the pale outer leaves. Put the cauliflower in a bowl, add the Digestive Spice and coconut oil and mix until well combined. Spread on a baking tray and roast for 30 minutes or until tender but still crunchy.

Transfer the warm roasted cauliflower to a large bowl and add the apple, grated celery, celery leaves, reserved cauliflower leaves and the cheese and gently toss to combine. Serve immediately.

+ **NOTE** Roquefort is a culinary delight that contains a number of essential vitamins and minerals, including vitamin D, which has anti-inflammatory properties and supports the immune system.

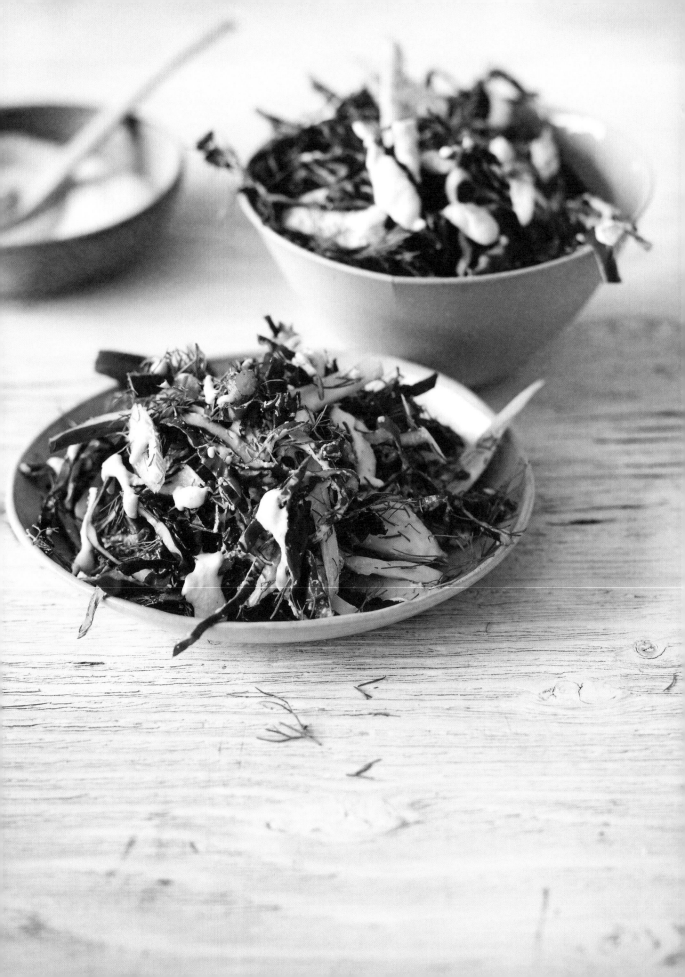

+ VEGETARIAN
+ VEGAN
+ GLUTEN-FREE
+ DAIRY-FREE
+ PALEO
+ RAW

PREP TIME:
15 minutes, plus
3 hours soaking

COOKING TIME:
Nil

FENNEL & PURPLE CABBAGE CASHEW SLAW

Slaw is great in this creamy dressing that is a nutritious alternative to mayonnaise dressings.

SERVES 4

400 g (14 oz) purple cabbage,
    finely shredded
3 fennel bulbs, tough outer leaves
    and core discarded, finely
    chopped, including the tops

DRESSING
310 g (11 oz/2 cups) raw cashews
60 ml (2 fl oz/¼ cup) olive oil
2 tablespoons grated fresh ginger
Juice of ½ lemon
2 teaspoons tamari (gluten-free
    soy sauce)
2 teaspoons thyme leaves
2 teaspoons oregano leaves
1 garlic clove
½ teaspoon salt

To make the dressing, soak the cashews in 1 litre (35 fl oz/4 cups) of water for 3 hours. Drain the cashews, then put them in a blender with the remaining dressing ingredients and 250 ml (9 fl oz/1 cup) of fresh water and blitz until smooth.

Put the cabbage and fennel into a large mixing bowl. Pour the cashew dressing over and mix until well coated. Serve immediately.

+ **NOTE** Purple cabbage is a delicious vegetable that is thought to assist in eye health and may also reduce the signs of ageing.

+ VEGETARIAN
+ VEGAN
+ GLUTEN-FREE
+ DAIRY-FREE
+ PALEO
+ RAW

PREP TIME:
15 minutes

COOKING TIME:
Nil

CAULIFLOWER TABOULEH

This tabouleh is grain-free and gluten-free, which makes it welcome at a barbecue or party where guests might have such dietary requirements. It's a lovely accompaniment to lamb or beef.

**SERVES 4 AS A SIDE /
MAKES 4 CUPS**

600 g (1 lb 5 oz) cauliflower
300 g (10½ oz/2 cups) cherry
    tomatoes, halved
1 small red (Spanish) onion,
    thinly sliced
20 g (¾ oz/1 cup) mint leaves,
    chopped
20 g (¾ oz/1 cup) flat-leaf (Italian)
    parsley, chopped
½ teaspoon salt
1 pinch freshly ground black
    pepper
40 g (1½ oz/¼ cup) pepitas
    (pumpkin seeds)

DRESSING
2 tablespoons olive oil
1 tablespoon apple cider vinegar
1 tablespoon lemon juice

Chop the cauliflower into bite-size pieces. Put them in a blender and process to a fine grain (a similar texture to couscous). Transfer to a medium bowl.

Add the cherry tomatoes, onion, mint, parsley, salt and pepper and mix well.

Just before serving, combine all of the dressing ingredients and toss through the salad until well coated.

Transfer to a serving dish and scatter the pepitas over.

+ **NOTE** Pepitas are the inner kernels of pumpkin seeds and contain zinc, magnesium and plant-based omega-3 fatty acids.

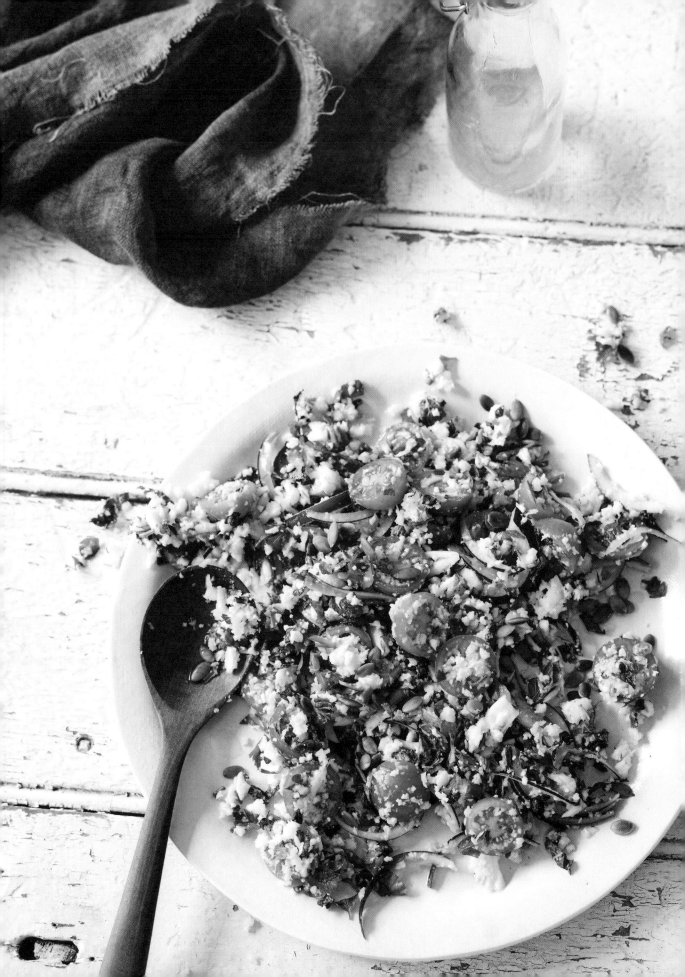

SOUPS

+ VEGETARIAN
+ VEGAN
+ GLUTEN-FREE
+ DAIRY-FREE
+ PALEO

PREP TIME:
10 minutes

COOKING TIME:
2½ hours

NOURISHING VEGIE & POTATO BROTH

This detox soup is a cleansing and nourishing combination of immune-boosting foods to help keep you healthy and glowing during a detox and beyond.

SERVES 4

3 celery stalks
3 carrots, unpeeled
3 sebago potatoes, scrubbed
1 tablespoon grated fresh ginger
2 tablespoons apple cider vinegar
1 bunch kale stalks
2 teaspoons pink Himalayan salt
1 teaspoon ground turmeric
1 teaspoon cayenne pepper
2 large pieces kombu
1 leek, halved and sliced
1 sweet potato (about 400 g/14 oz), scrubbed and quartered
100 g (3½ oz) dried shiitake mushrooms
1 tablespoon white (shiro) miso, to serve

Combine all of the ingredients in a large saucepan or stockpot. Add about 1 litre (35 fl oz/4 cups) of water or a little more if necessary, making sure the ingredients are well covered. Bring to the boil over high heat, then reduce the heat to the lowest setting possible and cook for 2 hours. Strain and discard the solids.

Serve ladled into four bowls, topped with a teaspoon of miso in each bowl.

Store in an airtight container in the fridge for up to 1 week or freeze in small containers for up to 3 months.

+ **NOTE** Potatoes are great in broths for gut health. Shiitake mushrooms provide immunity and miso is fermented for further gut-health benefits.

+ VEGETARIAN
+ VEGAN
+ GLUTEN-FREE
+ DAIRY-FREE

PREP TIME:
15 minutes

COOKING TIME:
30 minutes

CLEAN & GREEN SOUP

A bowl full of goodness that makes an ideal dinner option to cleanse your system without going hungry. The fennel aids digestion.

SERVES 4

500 g (1 lb 2 oz) broccoli, cut into
    florets, stalks reserved
4 fennel bulbs, halved
    lengthways, stalks reserved
1 tablespoon olive oil
½ teaspoon each salt and freshly
    ground black pepper
2 garlic cloves, finely chopped
12 large kale leaves, finely
    chopped, stalks discarded
    (about 12 cups)
1.5 litres (52 fl oz/6 cups) almond
    milk
2 tablespoons savoury yeast
    flakes
2 tablespoons tamari (gluten-free
    soy sauce)
Juice of 1–2 lemons

TOPPING CRISPS
1 tablespoon olive oil
2 garlic cloves, thinly sliced
1 tablespoon lemon zest
1 pinch salt

Preheat the oven to 180°C (350°F). Line a baking tray with baking paper and spread the broccoli florets and fennel on it. Drizzle with 2 teaspoons of the olive oil, season with the salt and pepper and roast for 12 minutes or until golden.

Meanwhile, to make the crisps, cut the fennel stalks and broccoli stalks into small cubes. Heat the olive oil in a frying pan over medium heat. Add the garlic slices and the chopped fennel and broccoli stalks and cook, tossing regularly for 5 minutes or until golden and crisp. Add the lemon zest and salt and remove from the heat.

Heat the remaining 2 teaspoons of olive oil in a saucepan over medium heat. Cook the chopped garlic and kale for 3 minutes or until soft. Add the oven-roasted vegies and the almond milk and simmer for 15 minutes or until all the vegetables are very tender. Remove from the heat, then stir in the savoury yeast flakes and tamari. Blend with a stick blender until smooth, then stir in lemon juice to taste.

To serve, ladle into four bowls and top with the crisps.

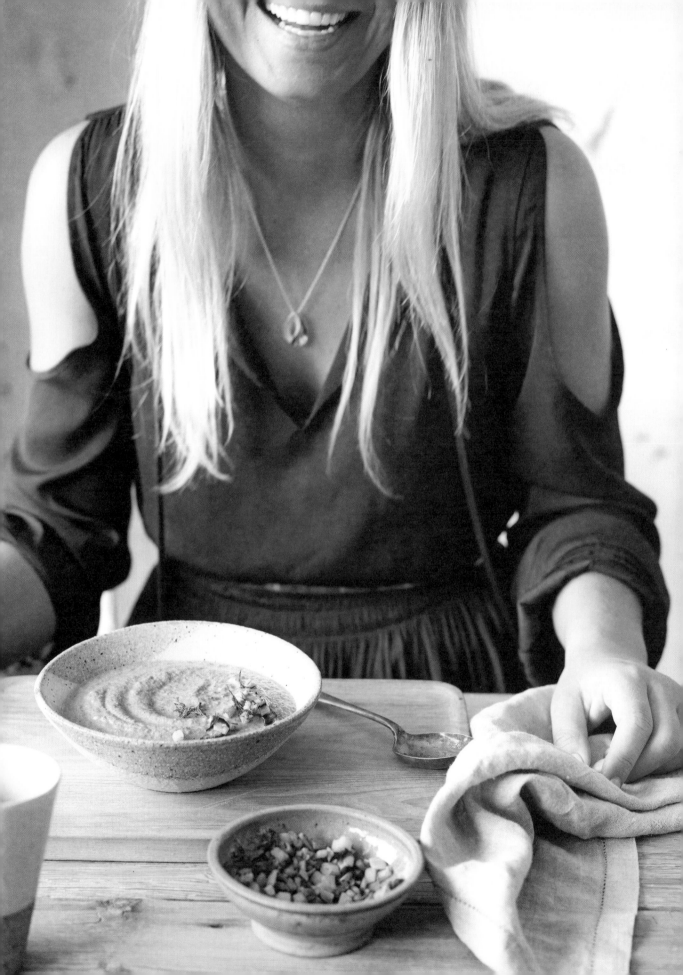

+ GLUTEN-FREE
+ DAIRY-FREE
+ PALEO

PREP TIME:
15 minutes

COOKING TIME:
20 minutes

GUT-HEALING IMMUNE-BOOSTING BROTH

Quick and easy healing broth for when you're feeling run down.

SERVES 4

1 litre (35 fl oz/4 cups) Nourishing Vegie & Potato Broth (see page 95) or Bone Broth (see facing page)
50 g (1¾ oz/¼ cup) peeled and thinly sliced fresh ginger
2 fresh long red chillies, seeded and thinly sliced
2 skinless chicken breast fillets, cut into 3 cm (1¼ inch) slices
2 carrots, thinly sliced
180 g (6¼ oz) snow peas (mangetout), trimmed
100 g (3½ oz) broccoli, cut into small florets
95 g (3¼ oz/⅓ cup) sheep's milk yoghurt
1 teaspoon apple cider vinegar
1 teaspoon ground turmeric
2 tablespoons chopped coriander (cilantro) leaves

Combine the broth, ginger and chilli in a saucepan over medium heat and bring to a simmer. Add the chicken, reduce the heat to low and gently poach for 10 minutes. Add the carrots, snow peas and broccoli and cook for another 3 minutes or until tender. Stir in the yoghurt, apple cider vinegar and turmeric and cook for another 2 minutes or until heated through. Ladle into four bowls and serve scattered with the coriander leaves.

+ **NOTE** The benefits of chicken soup combined with yoghurt is very healing. Our immune system starts in the gut so we need to look after its health.

PREP TIME:
10 minutes

COOKING TIME:
24 hours

BONE BROTH

Bone broth is simply amazing for your health! It is incredibly nutritious and health boosting while also very easy to make. I usually start just after I get home from work one day and the broth is ready the next day when I get home. I use it in curries and soups, for poaching meat, fish or vegies and for cooking rice or grains such as quinoa, freekeh and millet.

MAKES ABOUT 1–1.25 LITRES (35–44 FL OZ/4–5 CUPS)

1 tablespoon ghee
3 large grass-fed beef bones, about 600 g (1 lb 5 oz)
3 celery stalks
2 carrots
1 garlic clove, peeled and bruised
3 cm (1¼ inch) piece fresh ginger, unpeeled and bruised
2 tablespoons apple cider vinegar
30 g (1 oz/¼ cup) goji berries
1 bunch kale stalks
2 teaspoons pink Himalayan salt
6 black peppercorns
3 cm (1¼ inch) piece fresh turmeric, bruised

Heat the ghee in a large frying pan over high heat. Cook the bones until browned all over, then transfer to a large saucepan or stockpot. Add all of the remaining ingredients plus about 1.5 litres (52 fl oz/6 cups) of water, making sure everything is well covered. Bring to the boil over high heat, then reduce the heat to the lowest setting possible and simmer for 24 hours, skimming and topping up with extra water when necessary to keep the bones covered. The water should bubble very gently and not boil.

Strain the broth and discard the solids. Allow to cool slightly, then refrigerate until chilled. The chilled broth will have a layer of fat on the top. Skim this fat off and discard, then divide the broth into freezer bags or small airtight containers and refrigerate for up to 1 week or freeze for up to 3 months.

+ **NOTE** This broth includes immune-boosting foods to help keep you healthy, nourished and glowing. Avoid waste by using leftover kale stalks in this broth.

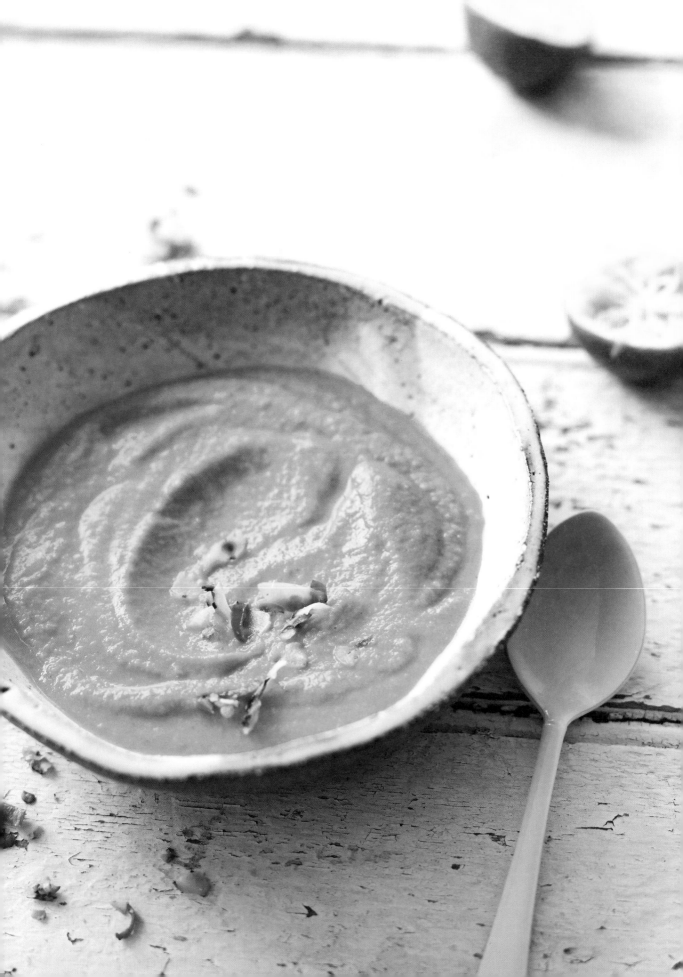

+ VEGETARIAN
+ VEGAN
+ GLUTEN-FREE
+ DAIRY-FREE

PREP TIME:
15 minutes

COOKING TIME:
20 minutes

SPICY GINGER & TOMATO SOUP

The vibrant colour of this rich antioxidant soup speaks for itself. You can really see the betacarotenoids in it.

SERVES 4

1 tablespoon coconut oil
1 large red (Spanish) onion, finely chopped
100 g (3½ oz/½ cup) coarsely chopped fresh ginger
6 carrots, chopped
2 x 400 g (14 oz) tins chopped tomatoes
375 ml (13 fl oz/1½ cups) tinned coconut milk
20 g (¾ oz/⅓ cup) chopped coriander (cilantro) leaves (optional)
1 lime

CRISPY TOPPING
2 teaspoons coconut oil
2 fresh long red chillies, sliced
2 teaspoons chopped fresh ginger
40 g (1½ oz/1 cup) coconut chips

Heat the coconut oil in a saucepan over medium heat. Add the onion and ginger and cook for 2–3 minutes until golden. Add the carrots, tomatoes and 375 ml (13 fl oz/1½ cups) of water and bring to the boil. Simmer for 15 minutes or until the carrots are very tender. Stir in the coconut milk, then remove from the heat. Using a stick blender, purée the soup until smooth. Season with salt and pepper.

Meanwhile, to make the crispy topping, heat the coconut oil in a frying pan over medium heat. Add the chilli, chopped ginger and coconut chips and stir for 5–6 minutes until crisp.

To serve, ladle the soup into four bowls, scatter with the crispy topping and coriander leaves (if using), then squeeze a lime over.

+ **NOTE** Tomatoes have the interesting attribute of being better for you when cooked. Cooking encourages the easier absorption of lycopene, a powerful antioxidant that may even have a role in cancer prevention.

KALE & BLACK RICE CONGEE

Congee is a rice soup or porridge that you can enjoy for breakfast, lunch and dinner. It's great during the cold autumn and winter months.

SERVES 4–6

1 tablespoon olive oil
1 large brown onion, finely chopped
2 garlic cloves, finely grated
2 tablespoons finely grated fresh ginger
600 g (1 lb 5 oz/3 cups) black rice
160 g (5¾ oz) shiitake or button mushrooms, sliced
4 large kale leaves, finely chopped, stalks discarded (about 4 cups)
290 g (10¼ oz/1 cup) white (shiro) miso
2 teaspoons salt
1 pinch freshly ground black pepper
6 sheets nori, torn into pieces
2 tablespoons tamari (gluten-free soy sauce)
2 tablespoons umeboshi (fermented Japanese plum) paste

Heat the olive oil in a large saucepan over medium heat. Cook the onion, garlic and ginger for 2–3 minutes until soft. Add the black rice and stir for 2 minutes or until well coated.

Add 2.5 litres (87 fl oz/10 cups) of water, bring to the boil, then reduce the heat to low and simmer for 30–40 minutes. Add the mushrooms and cook for another 10 minutes or until the rice is tender. Remove from the heat, stir in the kale and miso until well combined, then add the salt and pepper. Ladle into bowls and serve topped with the torn nori, tamari and umeboshi.

+ **NOTE** Black rice is rich in antioxidants, full of protein and high in iron, plus it delivers a delicious nutty flavour.

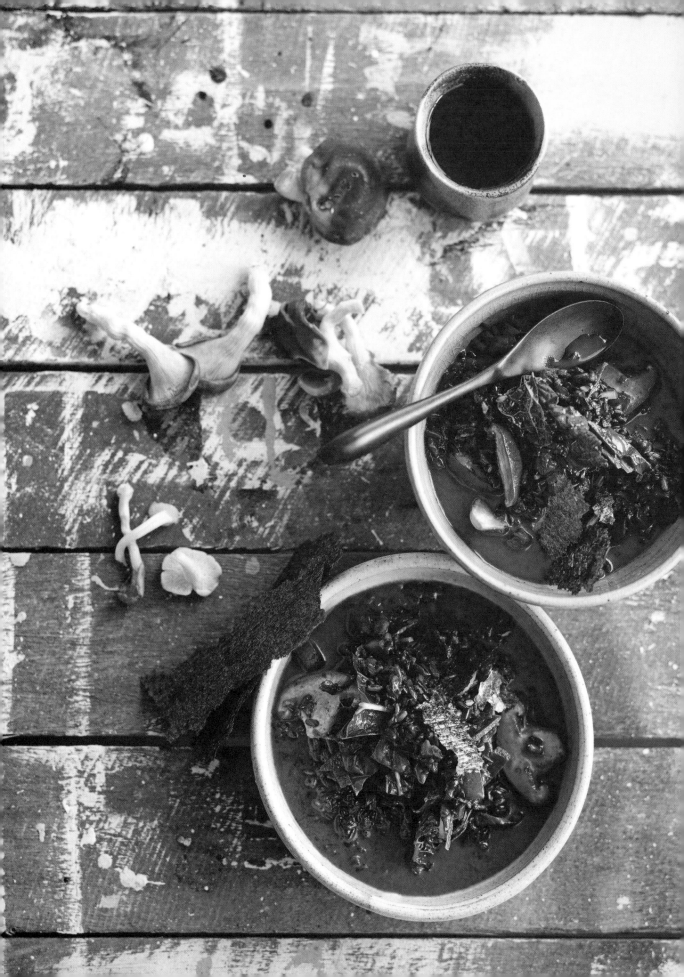

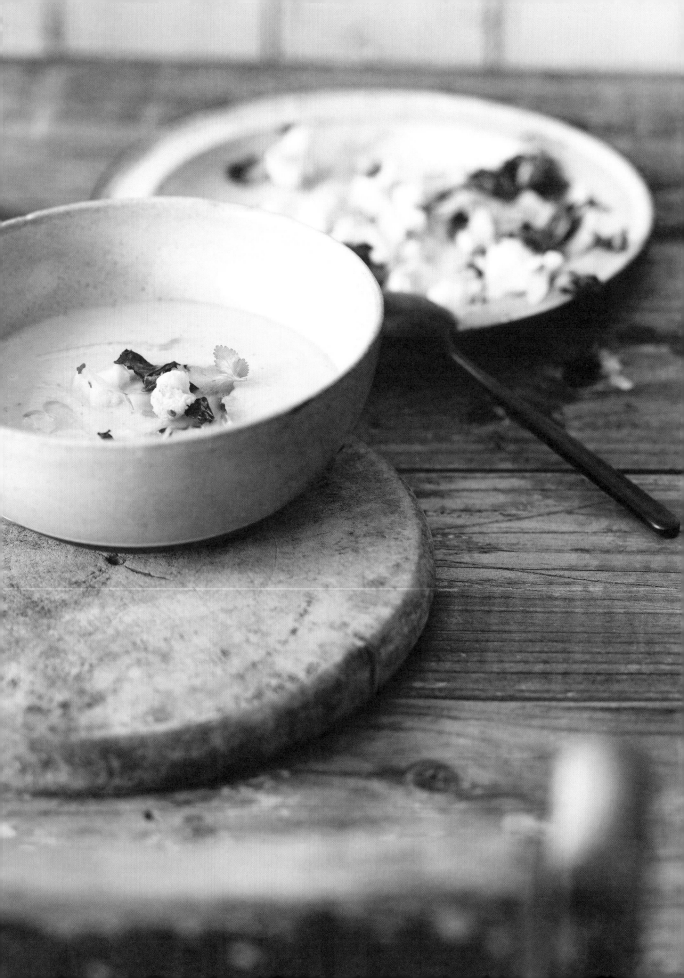

+ VEGETARIAN
+ VEGAN
+ GLUTEN-FREE
+ DAIRY-FREE
+ PALEO

PREP TIME:
15 minutes

COOKING TIME:
1 hour

TURMERIC CAULIFLOWER SOUP WITH CRISPY KALE TOPS

Cauliflower and ghee give this a luscious texture.

SERVES 4

1 cauliflower, about 800 g–1 kg
    (1 lb 12 oz–2 lb 4 oz)
2 tablespoons ghee
2 garlic cloves, thinly sliced
3 cm (1¼ inch) piece fresh
    turmeric, unpeeled, chopped
3 cm (1¼ inch) piece fresh ginger,
    unpeeled, chopped
1.5 litres (52 fl oz/6 cups) Bone
    Broth (see page 99) or
    Nourishing Vegie & Potato
    Broth (see page 95)
250 ml (9 fl oz/1 cup) coconut
    cream
½ teaspoon pink Himalayan salt
½ teaspoon freshly ground
    black pepper
Coriander (cilantro) leaves, to serve

TOPPING
1 large kale leaf, finely chopped,
    stalk removed (about 1 cup)
40 g (1½ oz/1 cup) coconut chips
2 tablespoons olive oil
1 teaspoon dried chilli flakes
¼ teaspoon salt

Coarsely chop the cauliflower and reserve 125 g (4½ oz/1 cup) of the small florets for the topping.

Heat the ghee in a large frying pan over medium heat. Cook the garlic for 1–2 minutes until fragrant, then add the chopped cauliflower, turmeric, ginger and the broth. Bring to the boil, then reduce the heat to low and simmer for 40 minutes. Stir in the coconut cream and cook gently for another 5 minutes or until just heated through: it's important not to heat the soup too much once the coconut cream has been added or it will curdle. Remove from the heat and use a stick blender to purée the soup until smooth. Season with the salt and pepper to taste.

Meanwhile, to make the topping, preheat the oven to 180°C (350°F). Line a baking tray with baking paper.

Combine the reserved cauliflower florets and all the topping ingredients on the prepared tray, mix well, then spread out and bake for 10 minutes or until lightly toasted.

To serve, ladle the soup into four bowls, scatter with the topping and garnish with coriander leaves.

LUNCH

+ VEGETARIAN
+ VEGAN
+ GLUTEN-FREE
+ DAIRY-FREE
+ PALEO

MISO MUSHROOM KELP NOODLES

*Fresh and great as a light meal or as a side,
you can add fish to this dish for an extra
boost of protein.*

SERVES 4

800 g (1 lb 12 oz) fresh kelp noodles
1 tablespoon coconut oil
600 g (1 lb 5 oz) assorted fresh
    mushrooms (oyster, enoki,
    button, swiss), sliced
400 ml (14 fl oz) tinned coconut
    milk
145 g (5¼ oz/½ cup) white (shiro)
    miso
350 g (12 oz/3½ cups) thinly sliced
    snow peas (mangetout)
300 g (10½ oz/5 cups) small
    broccoli florets
1 red capsicum (pepper), seeds
    and membrane removed,
    thinly sliced
4 spring onions (scallions), thinly
    sliced
Juice of 2 limes
2 teaspoons chopped coriander
    (cilantro) leaves
2 fresh long red chillies, seeded
    and finely chopped

Rinse the kelp noodles under cold running water, drain well and set aside.

Heat the coconut oil in a wide saucepan over medium heat. Add the mushrooms and stir for 3–4 minutes until beginning to soften. Add the coconut milk and miso and stir for another 2–3 minutes until well combined. Add the kelp noodles and stir for 3 minutes or until heated through. Remove the pan from the heat and stir in the snow peas, broccoli, capsicum, spring onion and lime juice, then season with salt and freshly ground black pepper. Divide among four bowls, scatter with coriander and chilli and serve.

+ **NOTE** Kelp noodles are high in minerals and low in kilojoules. Served hot or cold, they make a great substitute for regular pasta or noodles.

CAULI TUNA MELT

*This dish is great for lunch or dinner and
perfect to serve with any of the Chips Three Ways
(see pages 196–197).*

SERVES 2

185 g (6½ oz) tin tuna in oil,
    drained
2 tablespoons finely chopped dill,
    plus extra sprigs to serve
2 tablespoons Greek-style yoghurt
2 tablespoons grated mozzarella
    cheese, plus 45 g (1½ oz/⅓ cup)
    extra
Pickled Veg (see page 173),
    to serve

CAULIFLOWER FRITTER
200 g (7 oz/about 1½ cups)
    cauliflower, finely chopped
1 kale leaf, finely chopped, stalk
    removed (about 1 cup)
1 spring onion (scallion), finely
    chopped
2 eggs
1 tablespoon coconut flour
1 pinch each salt and freshly
    ground black pepper
1 tablespoon olive oil

Preheat the oven to 160°C (315°F) and the grill (broiler)
to medium–high.

To make the cauliflower fritter, combine all of the
ingredients except the olive oil in a mixing bowl. Heat
the olive oil on the stovetop in an ovenproof frying pan
over medium heat. Add the fritter mixture to the pan
and flatten with a spatula to cover the base of the pan
evenly. Reduce the heat to low and cook for 3 minutes,
then transfer to the oven and cook, uncovered, for
15 minutes.

Meanwhile, combine the tuna, dill, yoghurt and cheese
in a mixing bowl. Top the cooked fritter with the tuna
mixture and spread the extra cheese over the top. Cook
under the grill for 5–7 minutes until the cheese is melted
and golden.

Scatter extra dill sprigs over and cut into wedges.
Serve with Pickled Veg.

+ **NOTE** Tuna is high in good fats and omega 3,
    meaning it is has an anti-inflammatory effect. Choose
    sustainably caught tuna (caught with a line and pole).

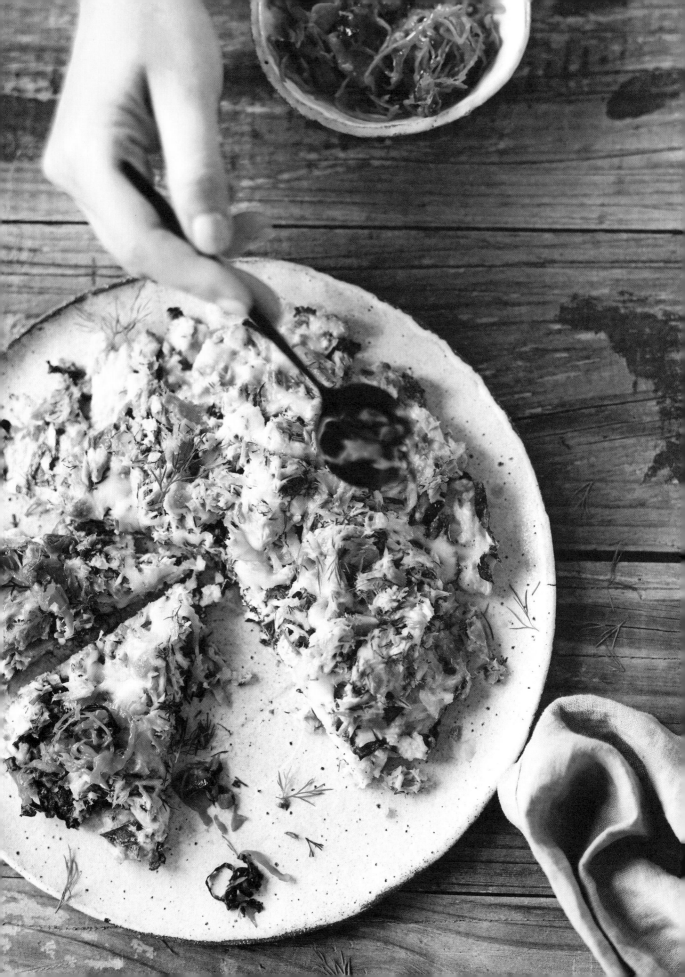

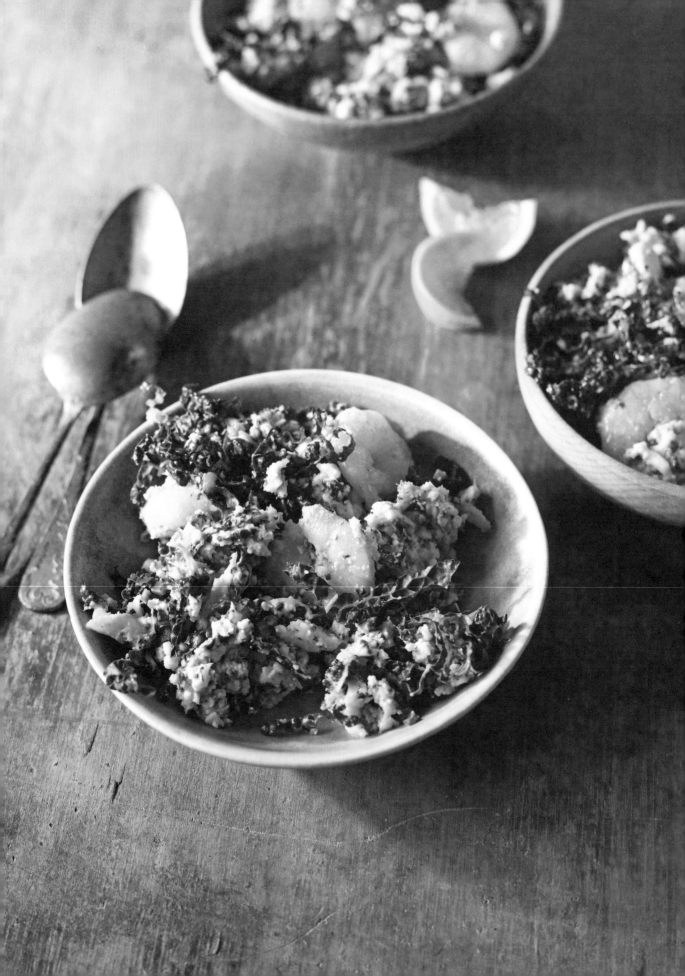

+ GLUTEN-FREE
+ DAIRY-FREE
+ PALEO

PREP TIME:
15 minutes

COOKING TIME:
10 minutes

PRAWN 'RISOTTO' WITH BROCCOLI CAULIFLOWER RICE

I love risotto but making it can be time consuming. Grain-free risotto, using cauliflower and broccoli, is easy, fast, nutritious and just as tasty. It's also easy on the digestive system.

SERVES 4

275 g (9¾ oz) broccoli
275 g (9¾ oz) cauliflower
1 teaspoon coconut oil
20 raw prawns (shrimp), peeled and deveined, tails removed
½ cup Activated Raw Kale Pesto (see page 60)
500 ml (17 fl oz/2 cups) tinned coconut milk
2 large kale leaves, finely chopped, stalks removed (about 2 cups)
15 g (½ oz/½ cup) coriander (cilantro) leaves (optional)
Lime wedges, to serve

Put the broccoli and cauliflower in a blender and blitz for 1 minute or until you get a rice-like consistency. Set aside.

Heat the coconut oil in a large frying pan over medium heat. Add the prawns and fry for 1 minute on each side or until they turn slightly pink. Add the pesto and coconut milk, bring to the boil, then reduce the heat to low and simmer for 3 minutes or until well combined and the pesto has melted through. Stir in the broccoli and cauliflower rice, season with salt and pepper, then add the kale and cook for another minute or two until just wilted. Divide among four bowls, scatter with the coriander (if using) and serve with lime wedges.

+ **NOTE** The activated raw kale pesto is the real hero ingredient here. The cashews add extra smoothness to the dish without using any cream.

+ GLUTEN-FREE
+ DAIRY-FREE
+ PALEO

PREP TIME:
15 minutes

COOKING TIME:
25 minutes

MATCHA DUKKAH CRUSTED SALMON

*Matcha gives the flavour a great lift and adds
an amazing bright green colour.*

SERVES 4

4 salmon fillets, about 170 g (6 oz)
 each, pinbones removed
¼ teaspoon pink Himalayan salt
1 teaspoon coconut oil
Spicy Cinnamon Sweet Potato
 Mash (see page 193), to serve

MATCHA DUKKAH
75 g (2¾ oz/½ cup) raw hazelnuts
70 g (2½ oz/½ cup) pistachios
1 tablespoon cumin seeds
1 tablespoon coriander seeds
1 tablespoon black sesame seeds
1 tablespoon white sesame seeds
1 tablespoon matcha (powdered
 green tea)

Preheat the oven to 150°C (300°F). To make the dukkah, put all of the ingredients, except the matcha, into a blender and blitz until coarsely chopped. Spread out on a baking tray and bake for 10 minutes or until just starting to colour. Remove from the oven and allow to cool on the tray, then stir through the matcha powder.

Lay the salmon flesh-side up on a plate and season with the salt. Spread a thin layer of dukkah evenly over the top of each piece and press firmly to help it stick.

Heat the coconut oil in a large nonstick frying pan over high heat. Place the salmon dukkah-side down in the pan and cook for 2 minutes or until the dukkah is golden. Reduce the heat to low, turn the fish over and cook for another 8–10 minutes until cooked to your liking. The cooking time will vary depending on the thickness of the fillets. Remove from the pan, stand for 2–3 minutes to rest, then serve with Spicy Cinnamon Sweet Potato Mash.

+ **NOTE** The dukkah recipe will make about 1 cup, which is more than you will need for this recipe, but you can keep the remainder for up to 2 months in an airtight container in the fridge. Use it as a crust on meat or fish, or simply serve it with sourdough bread and extra virgin olive oil for dipping.

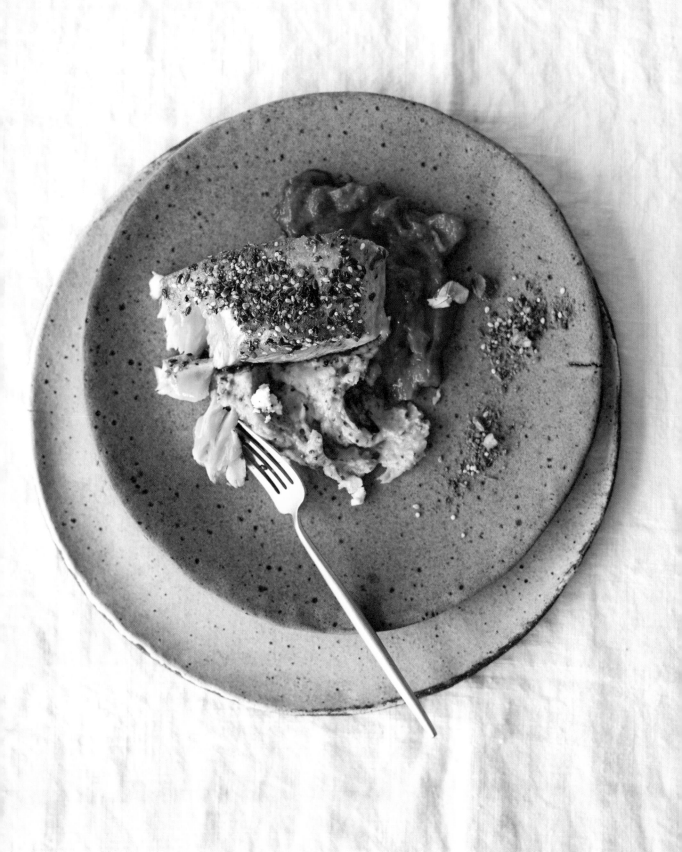

+ VEGETARIAN
+ VEGAN
+ GLUTEN-FREE
+ DAIRY-FREE
+ PALEO
+ RAW

PREP TIME:
1 hour, plus 2 hours chilling

COOKING TIME:
Nil

RAW DELICIOUS LASAGNE

Not your typical lasagne, this is nevertheless tasty, creamy and full of living enzymes. It goes really well with a peppery rocket (arugula) salad. It is one of our best-selling dishes and I often get asked for this recipe, so we've included it again here!

SERVES 6–8

40 g (1½ oz/¼ cup) linseeds (flaxseeds)

ZUCCHINI LAYER
4 zucchini (courgettes), tops trimmed
1 tablespoon dried oregano
2 tablespoons olive oil
2 pinches salt

WALNUT LAYER
40 g (1½ oz/⅓ cup) raw walnuts
155 g (5½ oz/1 cup) sundried tomatoes in oil, drained
2 teaspoons white (shiro) miso
2 teaspoons dried oregano
2 teaspoons dried sage
2 teaspoons tamari (gluten-free soy sauce)
¼ teaspoon cayenne pepper
1 tablespoon olive oil

TOMATO LAYER
110 g (3¾ oz/¾ cup) sundried tomatoes in oil, drained
2 dates, pitted
2 garlic cloves
2 tomatoes
1 teaspoon dried oregano
2 teaspoons olive oil

CHEESE LAYER
65 g (2½ oz) whole macadamia nuts (about 40)
40 g (1½ oz/¼ cup) pine nuts
2 tablespoons lemon juice
2 tablespoons savoury yeast flakes
1 tablespoon chopped flat-leaf (Italian) parsley
1 tablespoon thyme
1 pinch salt

PESTO LAYER
50 g (1¾ oz/1 cup firmly packed)
   basil leaves
125 ml (4 fl oz/½ cup) olive oil
40 g (1½ oz/¼ cup) pine nuts
2 garlic cloves
2 tablespoons lemon juice
¼ teaspoon pink Himalayan salt

To make the zucchini layer, use a vegetable peeler to slice the zucchini lengthways into thin ribbons. Put them in a bowl with the remaining ingredients and toss to combine well.

To make the remaining layers, put all of the ingredients for each layer into a blender and blend until well combined. Add 3–4 tablespoons of water to the cheese layer if necessary to thin out a little.

To assemble the lasagne, sprinkle half the linseeds over the base of a 36 x 24 cm (14½ x 9½ inch) lasagne dish or rectangular baking dish.

Lay a thin layer of zucchini strips (about one-fifth) over the base of the dish, then add all of the walnut mixture followed by half the tomato mixture. Top with another thin layer of zucchini, followed by all of the cheese mixture, another thin layer of zucchini, then the remaining tomato mixture. Finally, top with another thin layer of zucchini, all of the pesto, then the remaining zucchini. Sprinkle the remaining linseeds over the top.

Cover and refrigerate for 2 hours before serving.

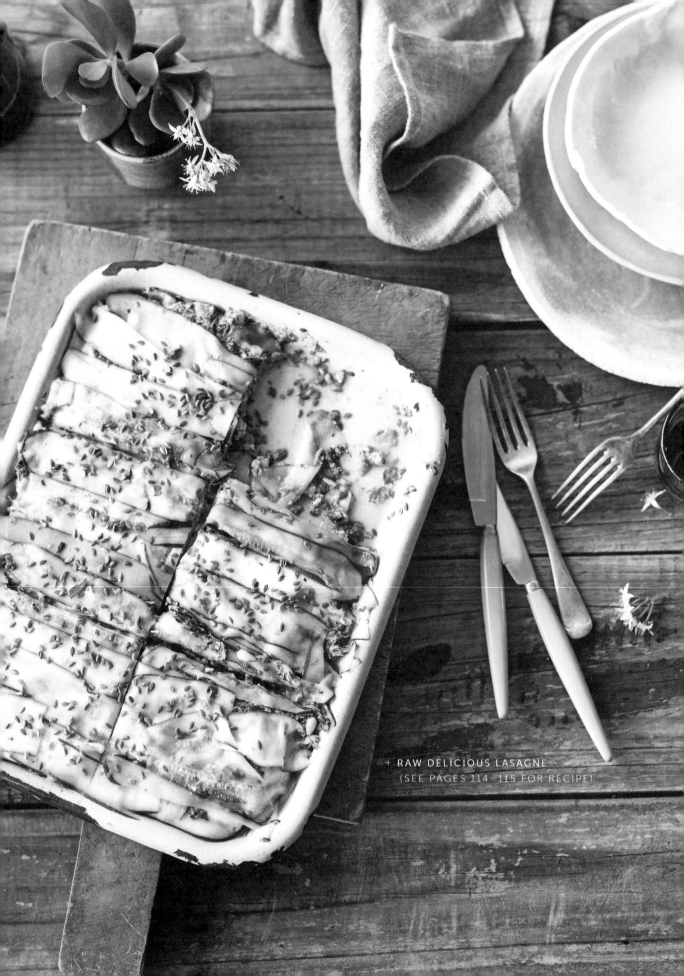

+ RAW DELICIOUS LASAGNE
(SEE PAGES 114–115 FOR RECIPE)

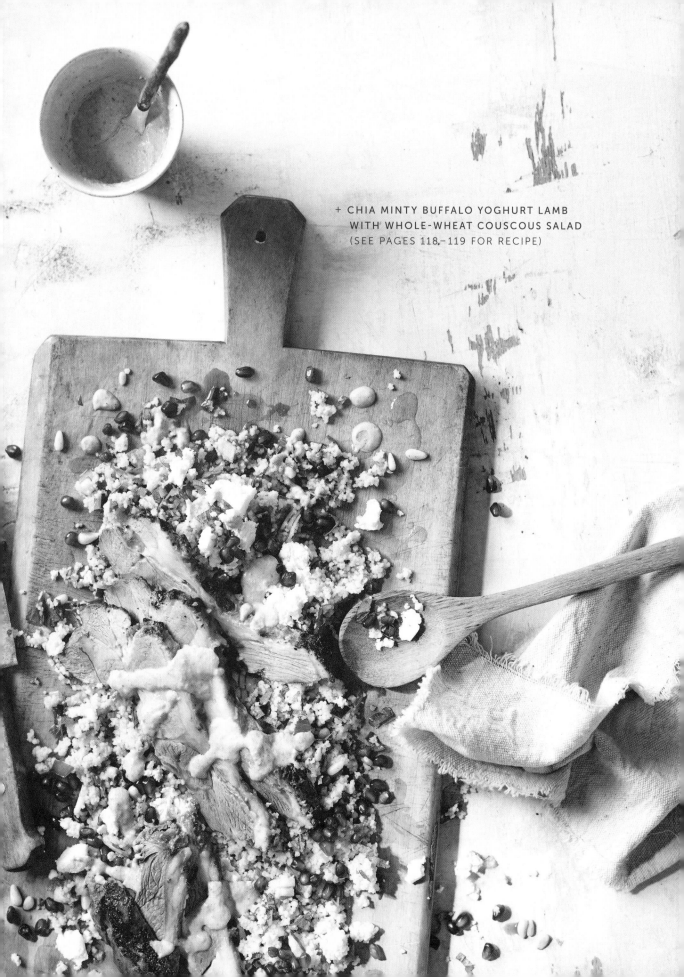

+ CHIA MINTY BUFFALO YOGHURT LAMB
WITH WHOLE-WHEAT COUSCOUS SALAD
(SEE PAGES 118–119 FOR RECIPE)

PREP TIME:
35 minutes, plus
1 hour marinating

COOKING TIME:
50 minutes

CHIA MINTY BUFFALO YOGHURT LAMB WITH WHOLE-WHEAT COUSCOUS SALAD

Great as a Sunday roast: something a little different to your traditional meal, but equally delicious.

SERVES 4

800–900 g (1 lb 12 oz–2 lb)
   butterflied lamb leg
2 tablespoons buffalo yoghurt
¼ teaspoon salt
2 teaspoons chia seeds

MARINADE
60 ml (2 fl oz/¼ cup) olive oil
20 g (¾ oz/small handful) rocket
   (arugula) leaves
2 garlic cloves
¼ teaspoon salt
Juice of 1 lemon
1 tablespoon dried oregano

YOGHURT COOKING SAUCE
260 g (9¼ oz/1 cup) buffalo
   yoghurt (or similar)
45 g (1½ oz/1 cup) baby spinach
   leaves
2 tablespoons mint leaves
2 tablespoons olive oil
¼ teaspoon salt

COUSCOUS SALAD
190 g (6¾ oz/1 cup) whole-wheat
   couscous
375 ml (13 fl oz/1½ cups) boiling
   water
155 g (5½ oz/1 cup) pine nuts,
   toasted
1 small red (Spanish) onion,
   finely chopped
30 g (1 oz/1 cup) coarsely chopped
   flat-leaf (Italian) parsley
2 tablespoons coarsely chopped
   mint leaves
60 ml (2 fl oz/¼ cup) olive oil
1 tablespoon apple cider vinegar
¼ teaspoon salt
130 g (4½ oz) feta cheese, cut
   into cubes
1 pomegranate, seeds removed
   (see note on page 81)

To make the marinade, combine all of the ingredients in a blender and blend until smooth. Transfer to a large bowl, add the lamb and turn to coat well, then cover and refrigerate for 1 hour.

Preheat the oven to 220°C (425°F).

Heat a large frying pan over high heat. Remove the lamb from the marinade (reserve the marinade) and cook the lamb for 2 minutes on each side or until golden. To make the yoghurt cooking sauce, combine all of the ingredients including the reserved marinade in a blender and blend until smooth. Transfer to a baking dish large enough to hold the lamb.

Put the lamb into the baking dish with the yoghurt sauce and turn to coat well. Cover the dish with foil and transfer to the oven. Reduce the oven temperature to 180°C (350°F) and bake for 35 minutes.

Meanwhile, to make the couscous salad, put the couscous in a heatproof bowl, pour the boiling water over, then cover and stand for 4–5 minutes until all of the water has been absorbed. Using a fork, fluff the couscous to separate the grains, then allow to cool. Stir through all of the remaining ingredients except the feta and pomegranate seeds. Set aside.

Remove the foil from the lamb, increase the oven temperature to 220°C (425°F) and bake for another 10 minutes or until the lamb is a deep golden colour. Remove the meat from the baking dish, reserve the dish and rest the meat for 5 minutes. Scrape all the juices from the reserved dish into a small blender. Add the buffalo yoghurt, salt, chia seeds and any resting juices from the meat and process to a smooth sauce.

To serve, spread the couscous salad on a serving platter and scatter with the feta and the pomegranate seeds. Thinly slice the lamb and lay the slices on top of the salad. Pour some of the sauce over and serve the remaining sauce in a small jug or bowl to pass separately.

+ **NOTE** Adding yoghurt to meats aids digestion. Buffalo yoghurt gives an extra-tasty flavour but you can use Greek-style, sheep's or goat's milk yoghurt or other natural yoghurts.

I have used chia seeds as a thickener for the sauce instead of adding flour, as chia seeds are high in good fats and fibre.

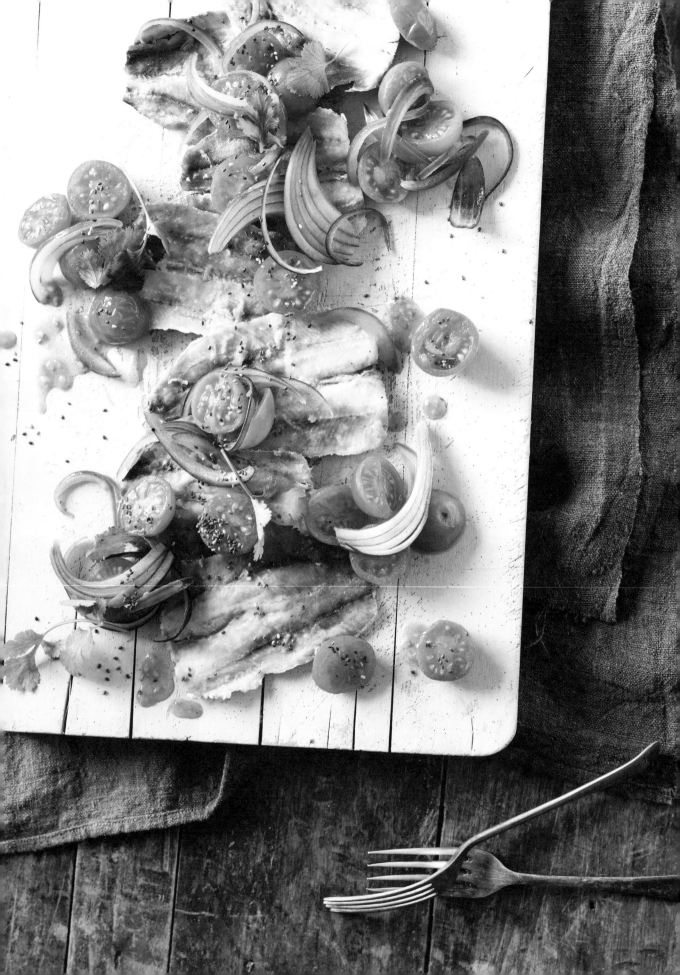

+ GLUTEN-FREE
+ DAIRY-FREE
+ PALEO

PREP TIME:
10 minutes

COOKING TIME:
10 minutes

LEMON SARDINES WITH CHERRY TOMATOES

I love tinned sardines in tomato sauce. Here I've recreated this favourite using fresh sardines and tomatoes, and it takes no time to make. It's great with a salad or served on Purple Seeded Bread (see page 31).

SERVES 4

12 fresh sardine fillets
Zest of 1 lemon
¼ teaspoon pink Himalayan salt
2 tablespoons olive oil
1 small red (Spanish) onion,
    thinly sliced
300 g (10½ oz/2 cups) cherry
    tomatoes, halved
1 tablespoon coriander (cilantro)
    leaves
2 teaspoons chia seeds
Lemon wedges, to serve

Preheat the oven to 180°C (350°F).

Lay the sardines skin-side down on a baking tray. Sprinkle with the lemon zest and salt, then drizzle with 1 tablespoon of the olive oil. Bake for 10 minutes or until just cooked through.

Meanwhile, heat the remaining olive oil in a frying pan over medium heat. Add the onion and cherry tomatoes and cook, stirring regularly, for 5 minutes or until the onion starts to soften. Remove from the heat and season with freshly ground black pepper.

Lay the sardines on a serving plate, spoon over the tomato mixture, then scatter with coriander leaves and chia seeds and serve immediately with lemon wedges.

+ **NOTE** Sardines are oily fish that are incredibly nutritious and, because they are small, they are a good clean option, packed with protein, and a rich source of omega-3 and vitamin D. It's useful to load up on these during winter when we see less of the sun.

PREP TIME:
15 minutes

COOKING TIME:
40 minutes

NUTRITIOUS MACARONI CHEESE

I love anything with cheese! This satisfying take on macaroni uses spelt or other wholemeal pasta, sweet potatoes and cauliflower.

SERVES 4

400 g (14 oz/about 1 large) sweet potato, peeled and chopped
600 g (1 lb 5 oz) dried spelt macaroni (or wholemeal wheat or gluten-free pasta)
300 g (10½ oz) cauliflower, cut into small florets
1 large kale leaf, finely chopped stalk removed (about 1 cup)
130 g (4½ oz/1 cup) crumbled feta cheese
300 g (10½ oz/3 cups) grated cheddar cheese

SAUCE
80 g (2¾ oz) unsalted butter
65 g (2½ oz/½ cup) spelt flour
420 ml (14½ fl oz/1⅔ cups) milk
400 ml (14 fl oz) tinned coconut milk
1 teaspoon salt
1 pinch freshly ground black pepper

Preheat the oven to 180°C (350°F).

Put the chopped sweet potato in a saucepan and cover with cold water. Bring to the boil over medium heat and cook for 15 minutes or until very soft. Drain, mash until smooth, then set aside.

Meanwhile, bring a large saucepan of lightly salted water to the boil. Add the pasta, stir well, then cook for 10–15 minutes until tender. Drain and return to the pan. Add the sweet potato mash and stir to combine.

To make the sauce, melt the butter in a small saucepan over low heat. When the butter has melted but not browned, add the flour and stir well with a wooden spoon until the mixture becomes thick and crumbly. Whisking continuously, gradually add the milk until smooth and well combined. Add the coconut milk, then simmer, whisking regularly, for 5 minutes or until the sauce is smooth and thick. Remove from the heat and season with the salt and pepper.

Stir the sauce into the pasta and sweet potato mixture and combine well. Add the cauliflower, kale, feta and 100 g (3½ oz/1 cup) of the grated cheddar and mix well. Spoon into a shallow 2 litre (70 fl oz/8 cup) capacity ovenproof dish, and scatter with the remaining cheddar. Bake for 15 minutes or until golden brown and crisp.

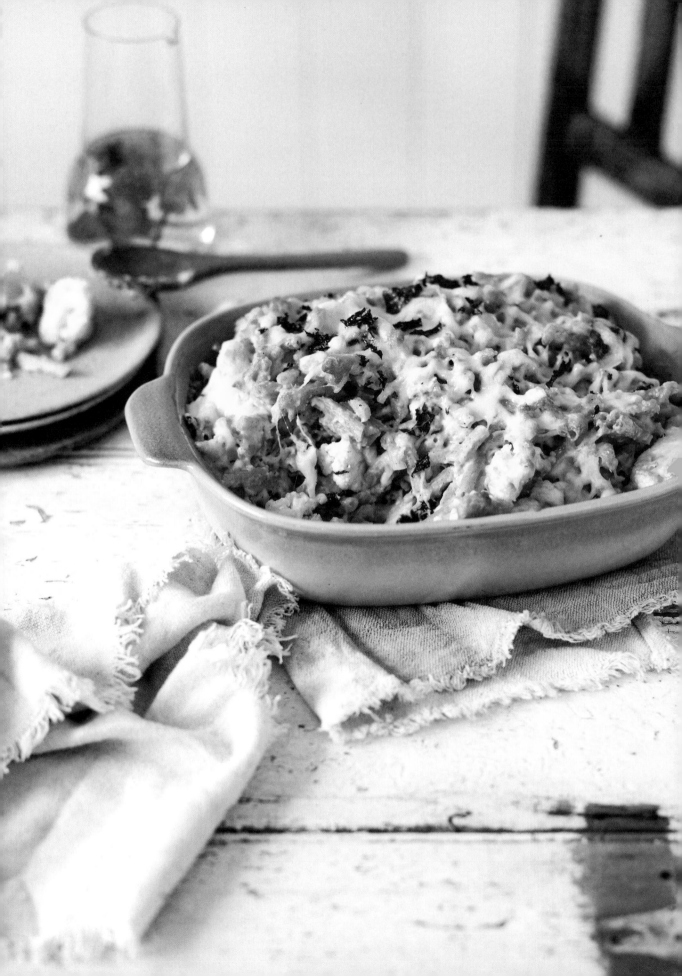

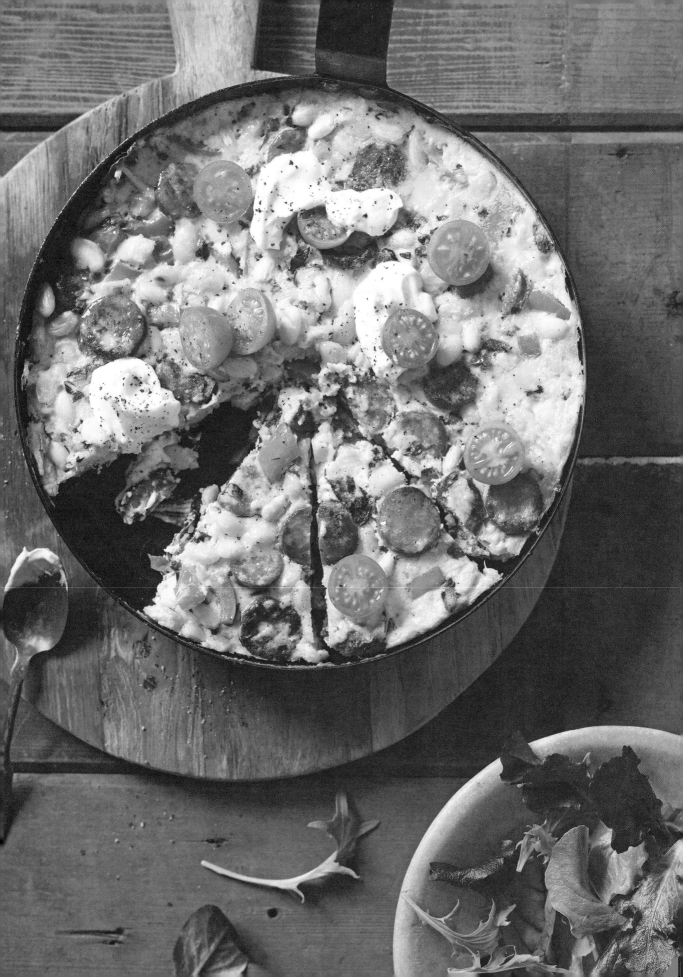

PREP TIME:
10 minutes

COOKING TIME:
30 minutes

CHORIZO WHITE BEAN FRITTATA

Frittatas are easy, quick and you can put almost anything in them, so they are perfect when you need to empty the fridge. Many frittata recipes call for cream; however, I always use goat's or sheep's milk yoghurt for boosted digestion.

SERVES 4

6 eggs
260 g (9¼ oz/1 cup) goat's or sheep's milk yoghurt
1 teaspoon each salt and freshly ground black pepper
½ teaspoon ground turmeric
250 g (9 oz/about 2) chorizo, chopped
1 silverbeet (Swiss chard) leaf, finely chopped, stalk removed (about 1 cup)
300 g (10½ oz/1 cup) cooked cannellini beans (see note)
½ red capsicum (pepper), seeds and membrane removed, finely chopped
15 g (½ oz/½ cup chopped flat-leaf (Italian) parsley
80 g (2¾ oz) cherry tomatoes, halved
150 g (5½ oz) fresh ricotta cheese
Salad greens, to serve

Preheat the oven to 180°C (350°F).

Put the eggs, yoghurt, salt, pepper and turmeric in a bowl and whisk to combine well, then set aside.

Heat a large ovenproof frying pan over medium heat. Add the chorizo and cook for 3–4 minutes until crisp. Add the silverbeet and cook for 2 minutes or until it starts to wilt. Add the beans, capsicum and parsley and stir to combine well. Pour the egg mixture over the top of the vegetables and cook, stirring occasionally, for 5 minutes or until the egg is starting to set.

Transfer the pan to the oven and bake for 10–15 minutes until just set. Remove from the oven and allow to cool to room temperature. Top with the cherry tomatoes and dollops of ricotta, season with cracked black pepper and serve with a green salad.

+ **NOTE** To cook cannellini beans, soak 200 g (7 oz/1 cup) of dried beans for at least 2 hours in water. Drain. Transfer to a saucepan with 750 ml (26 fl oz/3 cups) of fresh water and bring to the boil over high heat. Reduce the heat to low and simmer for 40 minutes or until tender. Drain. This makes 2 cups of cooked beans.

CRISPY COCONUT CHICKEN

*This is a crisp, refreshing and energising version
of chicken schnitzel. I like serving this with
Energising Nutty Sweet Potato Salad (see page 79),
but any of the salads in this book would work well.*

SERVES 4

3 eggs
80 g (2¾ oz/½ cup) white
    or brown rice flour
65 g (2½ oz/1 cup) shredded
    coconut
4 skinless chicken thigh fillets,
    about 800–900 g (1 lb 12 oz–
    2 lb) total
2 tablespoons coconut oil
1 teaspoon pink Himalayan salt

Whisk the eggs and flour in a bowl until well combined:
this method gives a crisp finish. Put the shredded
coconut in a separate bowl.

Working one at a time, dip each chicken thigh in the
egg mixture, allow the excess to drain off, then coat
in the coconut, pressing well to coat. Place on a plate.

Heat the coconut oil in a frying pan over high heat.
Sprinkle half the salt over the chicken pieces and put
them in the pan, salt-side down (the salt encourages
further crispiness to occur). Cook for 1 minute or until
crisp, then sprinkle the remaining salt over the chicken,
turn and cook on the other side for 1 minute or until
crisp. Reduce the heat to medium and cook for another
4 minutes on each side or until cooked through. Drain
on paper towel and serve warm.

+ **NOTE** I use shredded coconut as a substitute
    for breadcrumbs. It adds a beautiful nutty crunch
    to the chicken.

+ GLUTEN-FREE
+ DAIRY-FREE
+ PALEO

PREP TIME:
20 minutes

COOKING TIME:
10 minutes

KALE & LIME FISH CAKES

*These fish cakes are moist and bursting with
flavour and go well with your favourite dips.*

SERVES 4 (MAKES 4 PATTIES)

1 large kale leaf, finely chopped,
    stalk removed (about 1 cup)
360 g (12¾ oz) skinless firm
    white-fleshed fish fillets,
    chopped
2 teaspoons finely chopped
    fresh ginger
2 teaspoons finely chopped garlic
2 tablespoons chopped coriander
    (cilantro) leaves
½ teaspoon dried lemongrass
1 teaspoon lime zest
1 teaspoon lime juice
2 teaspoons red curry paste
1 tablespoon coconut flour
1 tablespoon coconut oil
Lime wedges and coriander
    (cilantro) sprigs, to serve

Put all of the ingredients, except the coconut oil, in a
blender and blitz until well combined. Using slightly
damp hands, divide the mixture into quarters and shape
into 2–3 cm (¾–1¼ inch) thick cakes.

Heat the coconut oil in a frying pan over medium-high
heat. Cook the fish cakes for 4 minutes on each side or
until golden. Drain on paper towel, then serve with lime
wedges and coriander sprigs.

───────

+ **NOTE** Lemongrass gives food or drink a lovely fresh
    flavour. You can buy it dried and powdered, or use the
    white part of fresh stems, thinly sliced.

+ GLUTEN-FREE
+ DAIRY-FREE
+ PALEO

PREP TIME:
20 minutes

COOKING TIME:
20 minutes

TURMERIC & LIME COCONUT BAKED SNAPPER

Golden, tasty and fresh, the turmeric, lime and coconut crumb works with just about any type of fish fillet.

SERVES 4

Coconut oil, for greasing
375 ml (13 fl oz/1½ cups) coconut cream
100 g (3½ oz/1 cup) almond meal
1 teaspoon ground turmeric
65 g (2½ oz/1 cup) shredded coconut
Zest of 2 limes
4 skinless snapper fillets, about 150 g (5½ oz) each, or other firm white-fleshed fish
¼ teaspoon salt
1 pinch freshly ground black pepper
Lime wedges and Coconut Cucumber Zoodles (see page 179), to serve

Preheat the oven to 180°C (350°F). Lightly grease a baking tray with coconut oil.

Using three shallow bowls, put the coconut cream in one, the combined almond meal and turmeric in another and the combined shredded coconut and lime zest in the third bowl.

Season the fish with the salt and pepper on both sides. Working with one fillet at a time, dip the fish in the coconut cream to coat well, then dip it in the almond meal and turmeric mixture, making sure the fish is well coated. Return it to the coconut cream and repeat the process. Finally dip it into the shredded coconut, pressing firmly so the mixture sticks to the fish. Lay it on the greased tray and repeat with the remaining fish fillets.

Bake for 20 minutes or until light golden and just cooked through. The cooking time will vary depending upon the thickness of the fish. Serve immediately with lime wedges and coconut cucumber zoodles.

+ **NOTE** Snapper is a good source of lean protein.

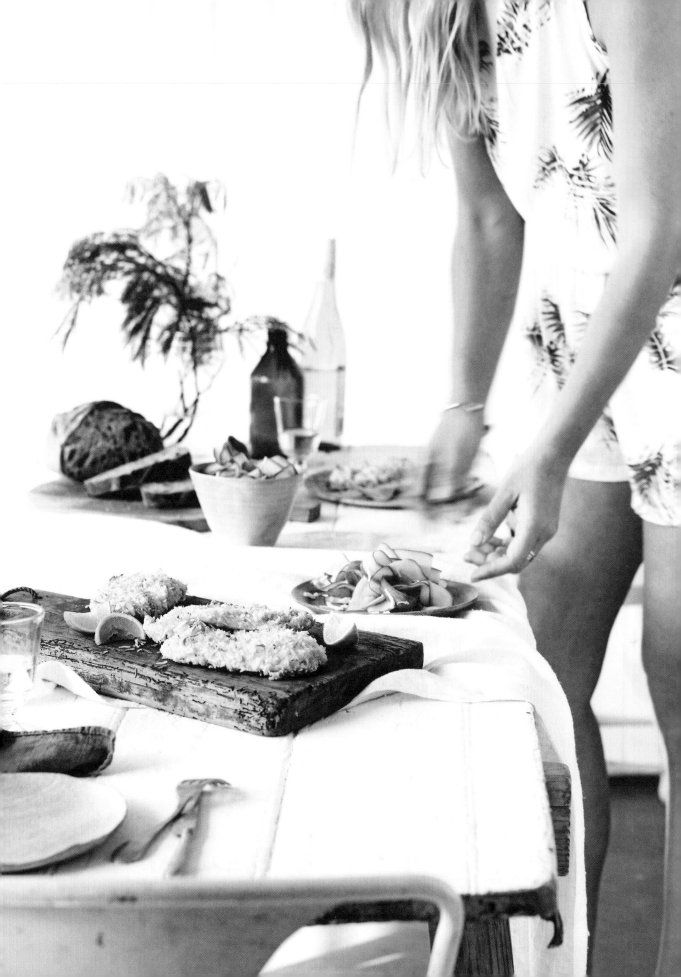

SPICED QUINOA FALAFEL

*I use quinoa for this gluten-free falafel.
This makes the dish higher in protein
than traditional falafel.*

MAKES 20

95 g (3¼ oz/½ cup) raw chickpeas,
    soaked overnight in cold water
100 g (3½ oz/½ cup) quinoa
1 large carrot, grated
2 spring onions (scallions),
    chopped
2 tablespoons chopped coriander
    (cilantro) leaves
2 teaspoons ground cumin
2 tablespoons ground turmeric
1 egg
2 garlic cloves, finely chopped
1½ tablespoons lemon juice
2 tablespoons tahini
½ teaspoon salt
1 pinch freshly ground black
    pepper
2 tablespoons chia seeds
2 tablespoons linseeds (flaxseeds)
Coconut oil, for frying

Drain the soaked chickpeas, put them in a saucepan and
cover with cold water. Bring to the boil over high heat,
then reduce the heat to low and simmer for 40 minutes
or until tender. Drain and set aside to cool.

Meanwhile, rinse the quinoa in a sieve under cold water.
Transfer to a saucepan, cover with water and bring to
the boil. Simmer over low heat for 15 minutes or until the
quinoa is light and fluffy. Drain well, then set aside to cool.

Put the carrot and spring onion in a blender and pulse
until chunky. Add the cooked chickpeas, half the cooked
quinoa and the coriander, cumin, turmeric, egg, garlic,
lemon juice, tahini, salt and pepper. Pulse again until
well combined but still chunky. Transfer to a large bowl,
stir through the remaining quinoa, then add the chia
seeds and linseeds and combine well.

Preheat the oven to 180°C (350°F).

Heat 1 tablespoon of coconut oil in a large nonstick
frying pan over medium–high heat. Work in batches:
shape tablespoons of the mixture into flat rounds and
cook for 3 minutes on each side or until golden. Put the
fried rounds on a nonstick baking tray and repeat with
the remaining mixture. Bake the falafel for 10 minutes,
then serve hot.

+ VEGETARIAN
+ VEGAN
+ GLUTEN-FREE
+ DAIRY-FREE

CHIA LENTIL BURGERS

*So easy to make, this vegan burger option
is just right for barbecues and casual
lunch parties.*

SERVES 4

410 g (14½ oz/2 cups) red lentils
50 g (1¾ oz/⅓ cup) coconut oil
*350 g (12 oz) sweet potato, peeled
   and grated*
1 large carrot, grated
1 tablespoon smoked paprika
1 tablespoon ground cumin
1 tablespoon ground coriander
1 teaspoon salt
*1 pinch freshly ground black
   pepper*
80 g (2¾ oz/¾ cup) almond meal
60 g (2¼ oz/⅓ cup) chia seeds
*20 g (¾ oz/⅓ cup) chopped
   coriander (cilantro) leaves*
Salad greens, to serve

Put the lentils in a saucepan and cover with cold water.
Bring to the boil over medium–high heat, then reduce
the heat to low and simmer for 15–20 minutes until soft.
Drain well, transfer to a mixing bowl and set aside until
cool enough to handle.

Meanwhile, heat 1 tablespoon of the coconut oil in
a frying pan over medium–high heat. Add the sweet
potato, carrot and spices and stir for 5 minutes or until
soft. Remove from the heat, add to the lentils and season
with the salt and pepper. Add the almond meal, chia
seeds and coriander and stir to combine well. Using
slightly damp hands, divide the mixture into quarters
and shape into patties about 2–3 cm (¾–1¼ inches) thick.

Heat the remaining coconut oil in a frying pan over
high heat. Cook the patties for 5 minutes on each side
or until golden. Serve with a green salad.

+ **NOTE** Lentils are an excellent source of plant-based
   protein, and so easy to cook. They are low in kilojoules
   and high in nutritional value.

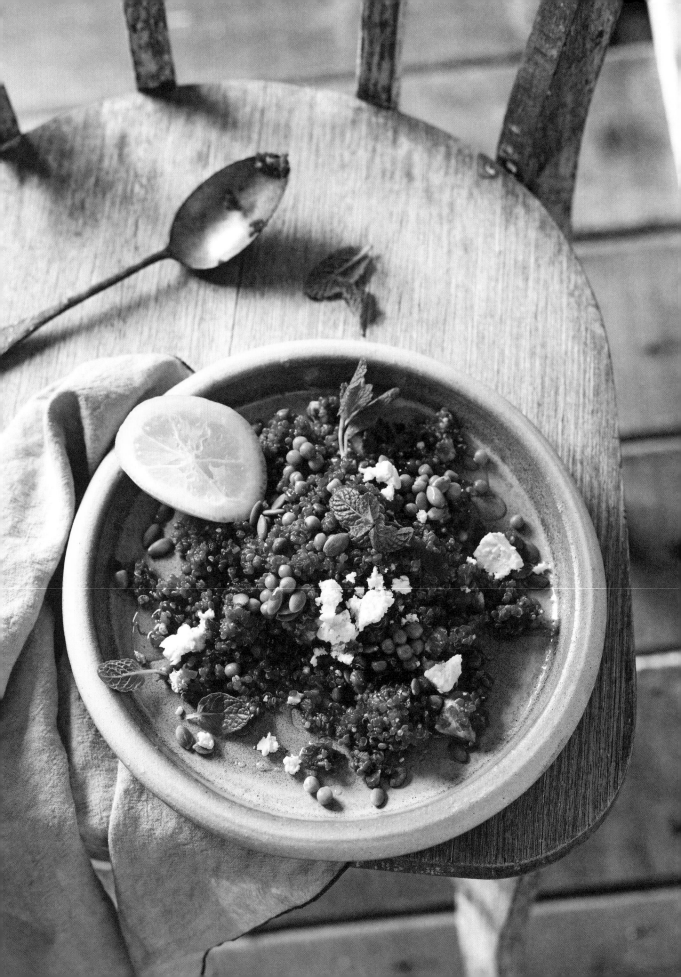

BEETROOT QUINOA 'RISOTTO'

This 'risotto' is great to have hot or cold. It lends itself to being eaten as a salad or a hot meal. The sweetness from the beetroot and saltiness from the feta is a great combo and it looks amazing with the beautiful vibrant colours.

SERVES 4

4 whole beetroot (beets), about 600 g (1 lb 5 oz), scrubbed
2 tablespoons olive oil
1 small onion, finely chopped
2 garlic cloves, finely grated
400 g (14 oz/2 cups) quinoa, soaked overnight and rinsed
195 g (6¾ oz) goat's feta cheese, crumbled
1 teaspoon salt
1 pinch freshly ground black pepper
280 g (10 oz/2 cups) frozen peas, defrosted
55 g (2 oz/⅓ cup) pepitas (pumpkin seeds)
10 g (⅜ oz/½ cup) mint leaves
Lemon wedges, to serve

Put the beetroot in a saucepan, cover with cold water and bring to the boil over high heat. Reduce the heat to low and simmer for 25 minutes or until a small knife withdraws easily when plunged into a beet. Drain, then put the beetroot in a blender and process until smooth.

Heat the olive oil in a large saucepan over medium heat. Add the onion and garlic and cook for 2–3 minutes until soft. Add the quinoa and stir until well combined. Add 1 litre (35 fl oz/4 cups) of water, about half a cup at a time, allowing each addition to be absorbed before adding the next. Continue until all the water is absorbed and the quinoa is cooked: it will take about 20 minutes. When cooked, add the beetroot purée and stir for 1–2 minutes until heated through.

Remove from the heat, stir through half the crumbled goat's feta, then season with the salt and pepper. Stir the peas through and stand for 1 minute, then divide among four serving bowls. Scatter with the pepitas, the remaining goat's feta and the mint and serve immediately with lemon wedges.

+ **NOTE** Beetroot is a good blood cleanser; in its strong colour, nature gives a visual clue that it's good for us.

TEFF GNOCCHI

*This is a traditional dish that I used to love
watching my grandma make. It is simple,
honest food with potatoes as the hero, but
I have combined it with contemporary ingredients
to give an extra boost of nutrients. This dish
is traditionally served with kefir for digestion.*

SERVES 4

1 teaspoon salt
1 kg (2 lb 4 oz) sheep's milk yoghurt
200 g (7 oz) sheep's feta cheese,
    crumbled
60 ml (2 fl oz/¼ cup) olive oil
150 g (5½ oz) bacon slices, finely
    chopped

GNOCCHI
580 g (1 lb 4½ oz) sebago potatoes
    (about 6 medium), scrubbed
300 g (10½ oz) cauliflower
280 g (10 oz/2 cups) teff flour
110 g (3¼ oz/⅔ cup) brown
    rice flour
120 g (4 oz/⅔ cup) sorghum flour
30 g (1 oz/¼ cup) tapioca starch
30 g (1 oz/¼ cup) potato starch
3 g (⅛ oz) xanthan gum
1 g (1⁄32 oz) guar gum
2 eggs

To make the gnocchi, put the potatoes in a saucepan of lightly salted cold water, bring to the boil over high heat, then reduce the heat to low and simmer until the potatoes are tender but not falling apart. Drain. When cool enough to handle, peel the potatoes and mash until smooth.

Meanwhile, cook the cauliflower in a separate saucepan of lightly salted boiling water until tender. Drain well, then mash until smooth.

Put all of the flours, starches and gums in a large bowl and stir to combine well. Add the mashed potato, mashed cauliflower and eggs, and season with salt and freshly ground black pepper. Stir until the mixture comes together, then knead until well combined and sticky.

Bring a large saucepan of water to the boil and add the salt.

Using slightly damp hands, shape heaped teaspoons of gnocchi dough into balls and place on a baking tray lined with baking paper. Drop the gnocchi into the boiling water and, as soon as they float to the top, remove with a slotted spoon, drain well and put them in a bowl.

Meanwhile, combine the yoghurt, sheep's feta and olive oil in a bowl and season with salt and pepper.

Cook the bacon in a large nonstick frying pan over medium heat until golden and crisp. Remove from the pan and set aside, then add the cooked gnocchi to the pan and shake for 3 minutes or until golden. Add the yoghurt mixture and cook for 3–4 minutes, shaking the pan regularly, until well combined and starting to thicken. Divide the gnocchi and sauce among four serving plates, scatter with the crisp bacon and serve immediately.

+ NOTE Teff is a little tiny grain that is almost starting to overtake quinoa in popularity. This little powerhouse is full of protein, has a low glycaemic index (GI) and is a great gluten-free option.

Xanthan and guar gums are natural thickening agents that are gluten free.

PREP TIME:
*15 minutes,
plus 48 hours
draining*

COOKING TIME:
25 minutes

GREEN PIZZA WITH SALAMI & GOLDEN LABNEH

*Labneh will keep in the fridge for up to a week.
If you don't use it all, pop the leftovers in a jar
and cover with your favourite flavour of olive oil.
I love mine with fresh chilli.*

SERVES 4

3 tablespoons Creamy Mint Pesto
    (see page 59)
12 thin slices spicy salami
Extra virgin olive oil, for drizzling
1 handful rocket (arugula) leaves

BASE
300 g (10½ oz) broccoli
45 g (1½ oz/1 cup) baby spinach
    leaves
15 g (½ oz/¼ cup firmly packed)
    basil leaves
150 g (5½ oz/1½ cups) almond meal
25 g (1 oz/¼ cup) finely grated
    parmesan cheese
2 eggs
½ teaspoon pink Himalayan salt

GOLDEN LABNEH
260 g (9¼ oz/1 cup) plain yoghurt
1 teaspoon ground turmeric
½ teaspoon salt

To make the labneh, mix all the ingredients together in a bowl. Line a sieve with muslin (cheesecloth) or 5 layers of damp paper towel. Put in the yoghurt mixture and twist the top tightly to enclose. Stand the sieve over a bowl in the fridge for 48 hours. Squeeze out excess liquid and store the labneh in the fridge until ready to use.

Preheat the oven to 180°C (350°F). Line a baking tray with baking paper.

To make the pizza base, put all of the ingredients in a blender with 125 ml (4 fl oz/½ cup) of water and blend until smooth. Spread the mixture out in a 1 cm (⅜ inch) thick round on the prepared tray. Bake for 20 minutes or until just cooked through.

Remove the base from the oven, top with dollops of pesto and the salami and bake for another 5 minutes. Remove from the oven, top with the golden labneh, then drizzle with olive oil and serve immediately, scattered with rocket.

+ **NOTE** Store leftover labneh in an airtight container, covered with olive oil, in the fridge for 5–7 days.

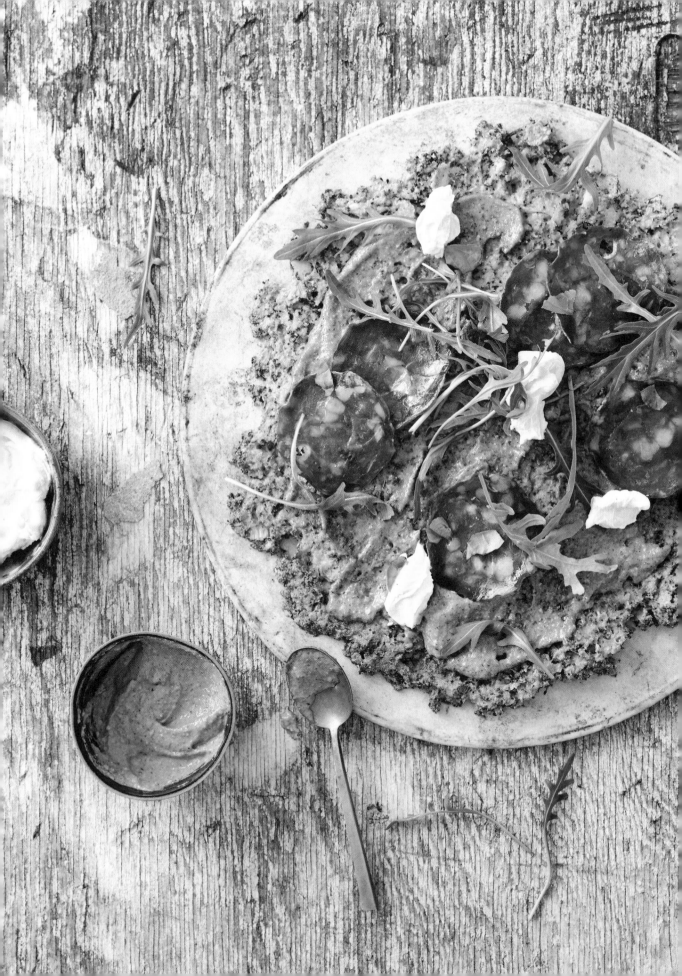

DINNER

+ GLUTEN-FREE
+ DAIRY-FREE
+ PALEO

PREP TIME:
30 minutes

COOKING TIME:
40 minutes

QUINOA MEATBALLS

These are a great favourite of mine: light and gluten free. I love having these with vegetable noodles.

SERVES 4

2 tablespoons olive oil
400 g (14 oz) tin chopped
    tomatoes
40 g (1½ oz/1 cup) torn basil
    leaves
Kale Pesto Zoodles (see page 178),
    to serve

MEATBALLS
750 g (1 lb 10 oz) minced (ground)
    beef
370 g (13 oz/2 cups) cooked quinoa
    (see note on page 12)
1 large brown onion, finely
    chopped
1 large carrot, grated
1 large zucchini (courgette),
    grated and excess liquid
    squeezed out
2 tablespoons tomato paste
    (concentrated purée)
60 ml (2 fl oz/¼ cup) tamari
    (gluten-free soy sauce)
3 teaspoons dried oregano
½ teaspoon salt
1 pinch freshly ground black
    pepper

Preheat the oven to 180°C (350°F).

To make the meatballs, combine all of the ingredients in a large bowl and use your hands to mix well. Shape tablespoons of the mixture into balls.

Heat the olive oil in a large frying pan over medium-high heat. Cook the meatballs for 5 minutes, turning regularly until golden. They do not have to be cooked through. Transfer the meatballs to a baking dish just large enough to fit them snugly in a single layer. Pour the chopped tomatoes over, then cover the dish with foil and bake for 25 minutes. Remove the foil and bake for another 10 minutes or until the meatballs are cooked through. Divide among four serving plates, scatter with the torn basil leaves and serve with Kale Pesto Zoodles.

+ **NOTE** Choose locally raised, hormone-free beef. I always try to go for grass-fed meat.

+ VEGETARIAN
+ VEGAN
+ GLUTEN-FREE
+ DAIRY-FREE

PREP TIME:
20 minutes, plus overnight soaking

COOKING TIME:
50 minutes

TURMERIC CHILLI BEANS & SWEET POTATOES

This is a vegetarian version of chilli-loaded potato skins.

SERVES 4

1 tablespoon olive oil
2 large sweet potatoes, about
  800 g (1 lb 12 oz), washed
2 avocados, halved lengthways,
  skin and stones discarded,
  coarsely chopped
15 g (½ oz/¼ cup) savoury yeast
  flakes
Juice of 1 lemon
Lime wedges, to serve

TURMERIC CHILLI BEAN MIX
260 g (9¼ oz) dried mixed beans
  (such as red kidney beans,
  cannellini and butter beans)
1 tablespoon olive oil
1 large onion, finely chopped
1 garlic clove, finely chopped
1 tablespoon dried chilli flakes or
  1 fresh long red chilli, finely
  chopped
1½ tablespoons ground turmeric
500 g (1 lb 2 oz/2 cups) chopped
  tinned tomatoes
1 tablespoon ground cinnamon

Soak the dried mixed beans overnight in cold water.

Preheat the oven to 200°C (400°F). Drizzle the olive oil over a small baking tray. Cut fine slices almost all of the way through the sweet potatoes, leaving the base intact. Put them, sliced-side up, on the tray and roast for 50 minutes, then reduce the heat to 180°C (350°F) and cook until tender. Set aside to cool slightly.

Meanwhile, to make the turmeric chilli bean mix, drain the soaked beans and put them in a saucepan with plenty of cold water. Bring to the boil over high heat, then reduce heat to low and simmer for 30 minutes or until tender. Remove from the heat and drain. Heat the oil in a frying pan over medium heat. Cook the onion and garlic for 2 minutes or until golden. Add the chilli and beans and cook for 5 minutes. Add the remaining ingredients, season with sea salt and black pepper and simmer for another 5 minutes or until the liquid has reduced and thickened. Remove from the heat.

Meanwhile, put the avocado in a bowl with the savoury yeast flakes and lemon juice. Season with salt and freshly ground black pepper and mash coarsely. Serve the potatoes with turmeric chilli beans, avocado mash and lime wedges.

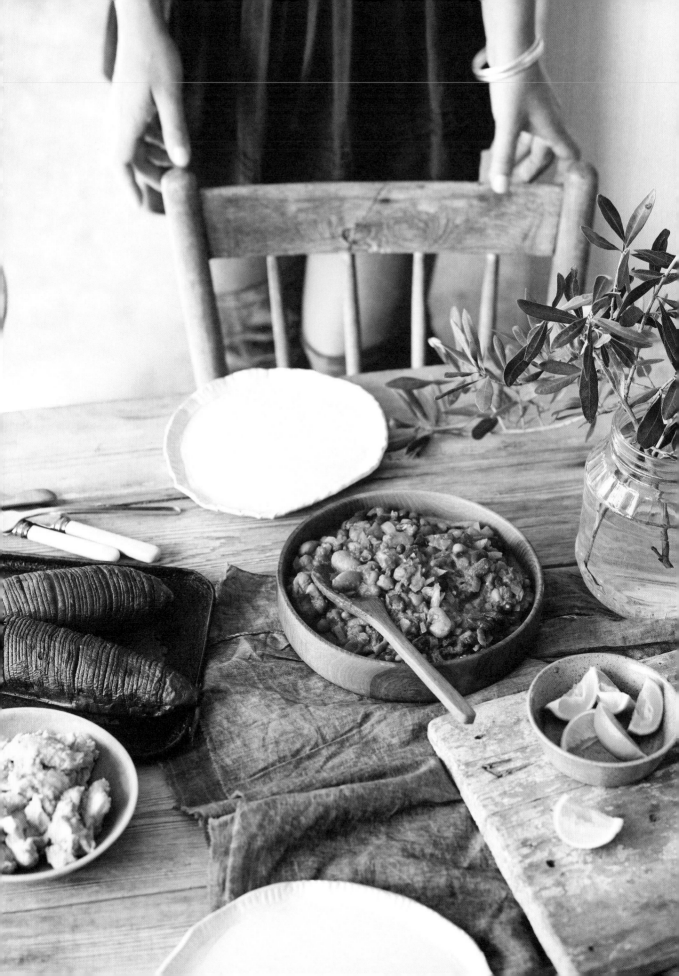

PREP TIME:
*35 minutes, plus
3 hours soaking*

COOKING TIME:
1½ hours

LAMB-STUFFED EGGPLANT WITH LEMON & WHITE BEAN TAHINI MASH

This dish looks fabulous on a platter when you are entertaining guests at a dinner party, plus it's easy to make and serve.

SERVES 4

3 teaspoons apple cider vinegar
2 eggplants (aubergines)
2 tablespoons olive oil
10 g (⅜ oz/⅓ cup) torn mint
    leaves

LEMON AND WHITE BEAN TAHINI MASH

120 g (4¼ oz/1 cup) dried white
    beans (see note)
1 garlic clove
125 ml (4 fl oz/½ cup) almond
    milk
90 g (3¼ oz/⅓ cup) tahini
2 tablespoons olive oil
Zest of 1 lemon
1½ tablespoons lemon juice

LAMB STUFFING

2 tablespoons olive oil
1 large brown onion, finely
    chopped
2 garlic cloves, finely chopped
500 g (1 lb 2 oz) minced (ground)
    lamb
250 g (9 oz/1 cup) crushed
    tomatoes
1 tablespoon dried basil
2 teaspoons dried rosemary
2 teaspoons dried oregano
2 teaspoons dried thyme
2 teaspoons smoked paprika
2 teaspoons ground fennel
½ teaspoon salt
½ teaspoon freshly ground
    black pepper

Soak the white beans in 250 ml (9 fl oz/1 cup) of water and the apple cider vinegar for 3 hours or overnight if time permits. Drain the beans, transfer to a saucepan, cover with cold water and bring to the boil over high heat. Reduce the heat to low and simmer for 1 hour or until tender. Drain and set aside.

Meanwhile, preheat the oven to 180°C (350°F). Cut the eggplants in half lengthways and place on a baking tray, cut-side up. Sprinkle with salt and drizzle with the olive oil, then bake for 30 minutes or until soft. Remove from the oven and leave on the tray until cool enough to handle.

To make the lamb mixture, heat the olive oil in a large frying pan over medium heat. Add the onion and garlic and cook for 3-4 minutes until golden. Add the lamb and cook, breaking up any lumps with a wooden spoon, for 5 minutes or until browned. Add the crushed tomatoes, herbs and spices and cook for another 5 minutes or until bubbling and slightly thickened, then remove from the heat.

Using a metal spoon, scoop the flesh from the eggplants, leaving a 1-2 cm (⅜-¾ inch) thick shell. Reserve the scooped out flesh and place the shells in a lightly greased baking dish. Divide the lamb mixture among the eggplant shells, then bake for 15-20 minutes or until they start to crisp up.

Meanwhile, to make the mash, put the garlic and almond milk in a saucepan and bring to the boil, then remove from the heat. Put the reserved eggplant flesh, the drained beans, tahini, olive oil, lemon zest and juice and 60 ml (2 fl oz/¼ cup) of water into a blender and process until well combined. Add the warm almond milk and blend until smooth. Season with salt and pepper.

To serve, divide the mash among four plates, top each with an eggplant half, scatter with the torn mint leaves and serve immediately.

+ NOTE You can use tinned beans instead of soaking dried beans if you prefer. Drain and rinse a 400 g (14 oz) tin of white beans.

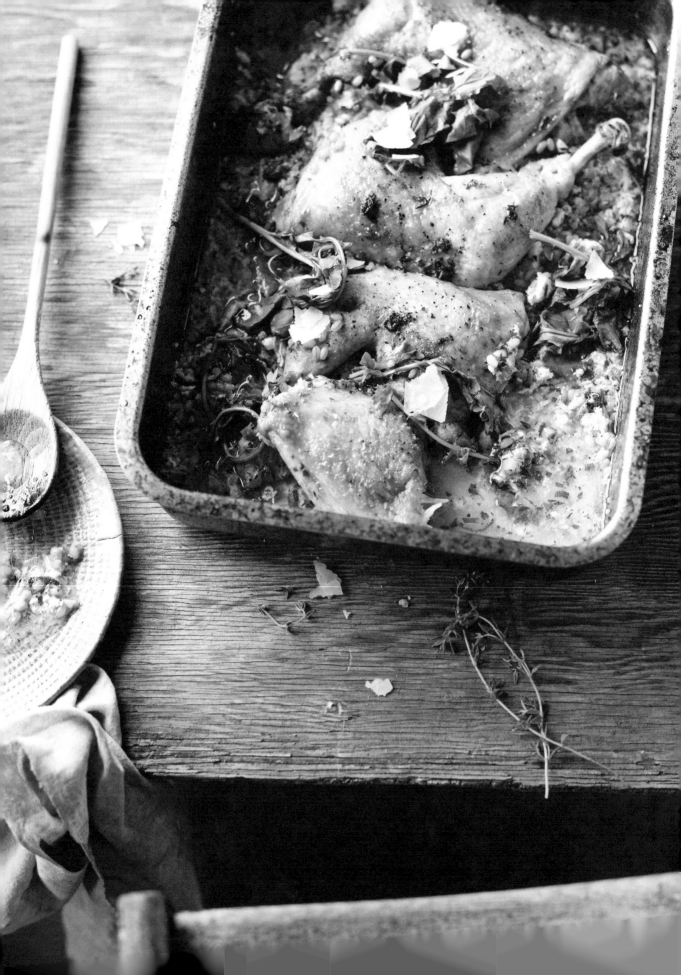

PREP TIME:
*20 minutes, plus
overnight soaking*

COOKING TIME:
1 hour

GREEK LEMON CHICKEN WITH FARRO & WILD ROCKET

In my teenage years, I spent my summer holidays in Greece where I got to eat the most incredible food, all made with quality seasonal ingredients. I loved the Greek lemon chicken soup: this dish is based on that flavour combination and served with farro and greens to make a substantial meal.

SERVES 4

200 g (7 oz/1 cup) farro (spelt)
60 ml (2 fl oz/¼ cup) olive oil
4 chicken Marylands (leg quarters), about 1.5 kg (3 lb 5 oz) total
⅓ cup garlic cloves, finely chopped
500 ml (17 fl oz/2 cups) Bone Broth (see page 99) or Nourishing Vegie & Potato Broth (see page 95)
80 ml (2½ fl oz/⅓ cup) lemon juice
½ teaspoon each salt and freshly ground black pepper
1½ tablespoons finely chopped sage leaves
¼ cup thyme leaves, plus a little extra to serve
1 tablespoon dried oregano
2 eggs, lightly beaten
2 large handfuls rocket (arugula)
1 teaspoon lemon zest
Extra virgin olive oil, for drizzling

Put the farro in a bowl, cover with cold water and soak overnight.

The following day, preheat the oven to 180°C (350°F).

Heat the olive oil in an ovenproof frying pan over high heat. Cook the chicken until golden all over. Remove and set aside. Add the garlic to the same pan and stir for 1–2 minutes until golden. Drain the farro and add to the pan with the chicken, broth and 250 ml (9 fl oz/1 cup) of water. Bring to the boil, then add the lemon juice, salt, pepper and herbs and stir to combine. Cover the pan with a lid or foil and bake for 40–50 minutes until the farro is tender.

Remove the pan from the oven and gently stir the egg through the farro. Bake, uncovered, for another 10 minutes or until the egg is creamy but not scrambled. Remove from the oven and fold the rocket and lemon zest through. Sprinkle with the extra thyme and a drizzle of olive oil and serve immediately.

+ GLUTEN-FREE
+ PALEO

PREP TIME:
10 minutes

COOKING TIME:
15 minutes

CHICKEN CARBONARA

This nutritious twist on a good old classic uses cauliflower and zucchini instead of pasta for a lighter dish, while goat's milk yoghurt reduces the amount of fat and also gives it a cheesy flavour.

SERVES 2

2 bacon slices, thinly sliced
1 garlic clove, thinly sliced
250 g (9 oz) chicken breast, thinly sliced
125 ml (4 fl oz/½ cup) pouring cream
130 g (4½ oz/½ cup) goat's milk yoghurt
1 tablespoon chopped thyme
125 g (4½ oz) cauliflower florets
1 large zucchini (courgette), grated
1 teaspoon chopped mint leaves
Lemon wedges, to serve

Heat a large frying pan over high heat. Add the bacon and garlic and cook for 2–3 minutes until golden. Add the chicken breast and stir-fry until golden: it doesn't have to be cooked through.

Remove the chicken from the pan and set aside, then add the cream, yoghurt and thyme and cook for 5 minutes or until slightly thickened. Add the cauliflower and cook for another 3 minutes or until tender, then return the chicken to the pan and simmer until just cooked through.

Stir in the zucchini, season with salt and freshly ground black pepper and cook for another minute or until heated through. Divide between two bowls, scatter with the mint and serve immediately with lemon wedges.

SHEPHERD'S PIE WITH LENTILS

This recipe has a few unusual twists to boost nutrition.

SERVES 6

150 g (5½ oz/⅔ cup) green lentils
1 tablespoon olive oil
1 onion, finely chopped
2 garlic cloves, finely chopped
1 spring onion (scallion), chopped
10 g (⅜ oz/⅓ cup) chopped parsley
2 teaspoons chopped basil
2 teaspoons dried oregano
500 g (1 lb 2 oz) minced (ground) lamb
2 carrots, thinly sliced
250 ml (9 fl oz/1 cup) tomato passata (puréed tomatoes)
2 teaspoons smoked paprika
1 tablespoon tamari
1 tablespoon brown rice miso
250 ml (9 fl oz/1 cup) hot water
45 g (1½ oz/¼ cup) brown rice flour
4 dried bay leaves
1 large kale leaf, thinly sliced, stalk removed (about 1 cup)

CAULI AND PEA TOPPING
500 g (1 lb 2 oz) cauliflower florets
280 g (10 oz/2 cups) peas
10 g (⅜ oz/½ cup) mint leaves
90 g (3¼ oz/2 cups) spinach leaves
130 g (4½ oz/½ cup) Greek-style yoghurt
1½ tablespoons olive oil
50 g (1¾ oz/½ cup) grated parmesan cheese

Rinse the lentils, then put them in a saucepan with 1.25 litres (44 fl oz/5 cups) of lightly salted water. Bring to the boil over high heat, then reduce heat to medium and simmer for 15 minutes or until tender. Drain and set aside.

Preheat the oven to 180°C (350°F).

Heat the olive oil in a large frying pan over medium heat. Add the onion, garlic, spring onion, parsley, basil and oregano and stir for 2 minutes or until the translucent. Increase the heat to high, add the lamb mince and cook, breaking up any lumps with a wooden spoon, for 5 minutes or until browned. Add the carrot, passata, paprika and tamari and stir to combine well. Stir the miso into the hot water until dissolved, then add to the pan with the rice flour, bay leaves and cooked lentils. Stir to combine, then reduce the heat to low and cook, stirring often, for 20 minutes or until thickened. Stir in the kale, season with salt and pepper, then remove from the heat.

Meanwhile, to make the topping, cook the cauliflower in lightly salted boiling water for 10 minutes. Add the peas and cook for another 5 minutes. Drain well, then transfer to a blender with the mint, spinach, yoghurt and olive oil and process until coarsely chopped.

Spoon the lamb mixture into a 25 cm (10 inch) round baking dish. Top with the cauliflower and pea topping and bake for 30 minutes. Sprinkle with the parmesan and a little freshly ground black pepper and bake for another 15 minutes or until golden and bubbling.

MUSHROOM & SILVERBEET AMARANTH 'RISOTTO'

This 'risotto', made from amaranth seeds instead of rice, is quick and easy. You don't need to stir it as much as rice and it has a great nutty flavour.

SERVES 4

420 g (15 oz/2 cups) amaranth seeds
1 tablespoon apple cider vinegar
30 g (1 oz/1 cup) dried shiitake mushrooms
30 g (1 oz/1 cup) dried porcini mushrooms
625 ml (21½ fl oz/2½ cups) boiling water
125 ml (4 fl oz/½ cup) almond milk
50 g (1¾ oz/½ cup) almond meal
1 tablespoon olive oil
1 garlic clove, finely chopped
120 g (4¼ oz) French shallots, finely chopped
160 g (5¾ oz) button mushrooms, chopped
1 teaspoon each salt and freshly ground black pepper
2 teaspoons chopped thyme
50 g (1¾ oz/½ cup) finely grated parmesan cheese, plus extra to serve
140 g (5 oz) silverbeet (Swiss chard) leaves, chopped
Extra virgin olive oil, for drizzling
Dried chilli flakes (optional)

Put the amaranth seeds in a large bowl, add the vinegar and 1 litre (35 fl oz/4 cups) of water, then soak overnight.

Put the shiitake and porcini mushrooms in a bowl with the boiling water and soak for 15 minutes or until soft. Drain, reserving the soaking water, and coarsely chop the mushrooms. Pour the soaking water into a jug, add the almond milk and almond meal and whisk with a fork until well combined.

Drain the soaked amaranth seeds through a fine sieve and rinse well.

Heat the olive oil in a saucepan over medium heat. Add the garlic and shallots and cook for 3 minutes or until golden. Add the amaranth and stir for 5 minutes or until the colour starts to change. Add the almond milk mixture and stir for 2 minutes or until well combined. Stir in 500 ml (17 fl oz/2 cups) of water, then add the soaked and fresh mushrooms, salt, pepper and thyme. Cover and cook, stirring occasionally, for 10 minutes. Stir through the parmesan and silverbeet and cook for another 5 minutes or until the silverbeet has wilted.

Spoon the risotto into four bowls. Drizzle with extra virgin olive oil, sprinkle with a little extra parmesan and the chilli flakes, if using, and serve immediately.

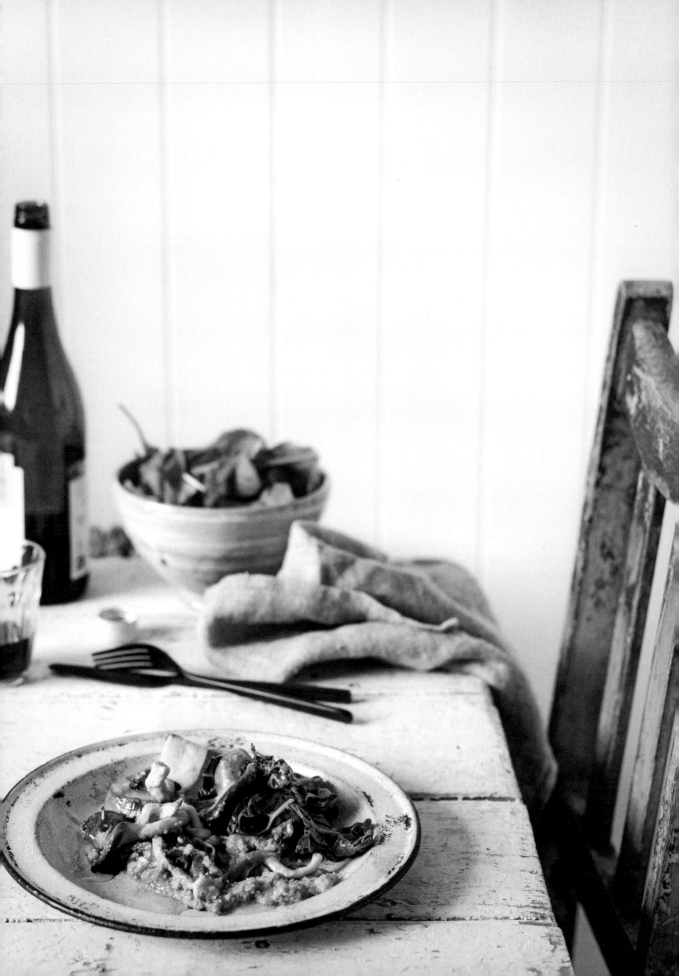

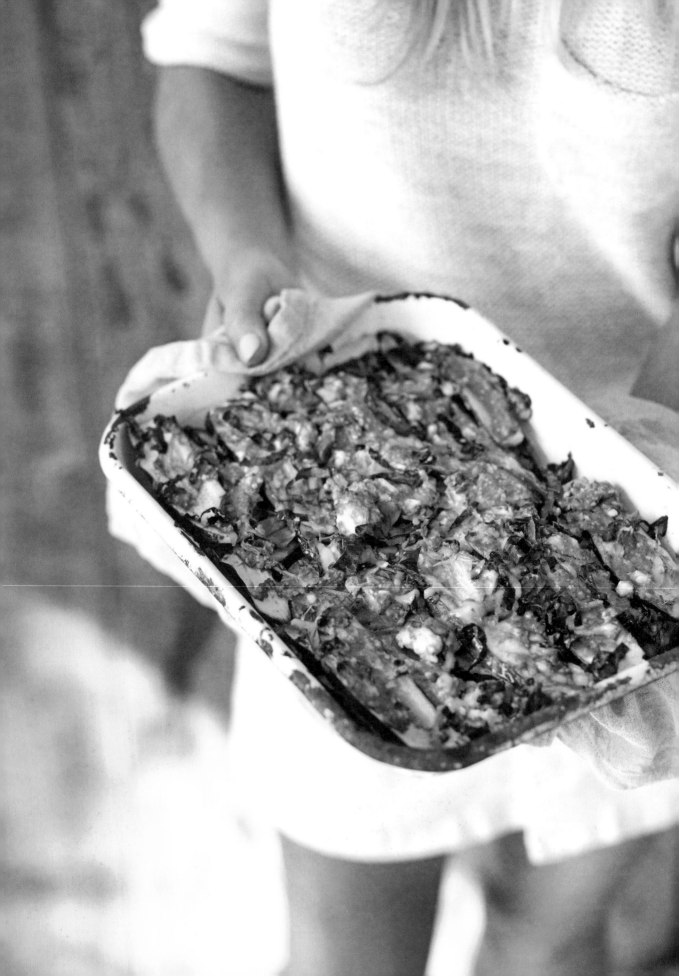

+ VEGETARIAN
+ GLUTEN-FREE

GREEN LASAGNE

This lasagne is quick, clean and green: it celebrates all the goodness, with healthy fats and a blast of calcium all in one dish.

SERVES 6

3 zucchini (courgettes)
1 eggplant (aubergine)
280 g (10 oz) cottage cheese
200 g (7 oz) feta cheese, crumbled
150 g (5½ oz/1½ cups) grated
    pecorino cheese
1 teaspoon spirulina powder
2 tablespoons chopped basil
1 tablespoon finely chopped
    garlic
125 ml (4 fl oz/½ cup) kefir,
    or use plain yoghurt
2 tablespoons olive oil
90 g (3¼ oz/2 cups) baby spinach
    leaves

KALE TOPPING
1 large kale leaf, chopped, stalk
    removed (about 1 cup)
½ teaspoon chilli flakes
1 tablespoon grated pecorino
    cheese
1 tablespoon olive oil

Preheat the oven to 180°C (350°F).

Slice the zucchini lengthways into 5 mm (¼ inch) strips and the eggplant into 5 mm (¼ inch) rounds.

Put the cottage cheese, feta, 100 g (3½ oz/1 cup) of the pecorino, the spirulina powder, basil, garlic and kefir in a bowl and combine well.

Pour the olive oil in a thin layer over the base of a 1.5 litre (52 fl oz/6 cup) capacity rectangular baking dish. Cover the base with half the eggplant and season with salt. Spread with half the cheese mixture, then cover with half the spinach leaves, followed by half the zucchini. Repeat the layers. Bake for 40 minutes or until cooked through and bubbling.

Meanwhile, combine all of the kale topping ingredients in a bowl.

Remove the lasagne from the oven and increase the temperature to 250°C (500°F). Top the lasagne with the kale mixture and bake for another 10 minutes or until the kale is crisp. Serve warm.

+ **NOTE** Spirulina is rich in antioxidants, vitamins, minerals, amino acids and easily digested iron.

+ GLUTEN-FREE
+ DAIRY-FREE
+ PALEO

PREP TIME:
15 minutes

COOKING TIME:
20 minutes

LEMON & THYME MACADAMIA CRUSTED FISH

This crusted fish with macadamias is a great combination with thyme. It's high in protein and needs no breadcrumbs.

SERVES 4

310 g (11 oz/2 cups) raw
    macadamia nuts
2 teaspoons finely grated
    lemon zest
2 teaspoons chopped garlic
⅓ cup chopped thyme leaves
1 pinch each salt and freshly
    ground black pepper
1 tablespoon melted coconut oil
250 g (9 oz) skinless firm white-
    fleshed fish fillets (such as
    ling, snapper or barramundi)

Preheat the oven to 180°C (350°F). Lightly grease a baking tray.

Put the macadamia nuts, lemon zest, garlic, thyme, salt and pepper in a blender and process until coarsely chopped. Transfer to a bowl and stir the melted coconut oil through.

Lay the fish fillets on the prepared baking tray. Spread the macadamia mixture over the fish and press lightly. Bake for 15–20 minutes until just cooked through.

+ **NOTE** Macadamias, native to Australia, are an excellent source of minerals such as calcium, iron and magnesium.

+ VEGETARIAN
+ VEGAN
+ GLUTEN-FREE
+ DAIRY-FREE

PREP TIME:
15 minutes

COOKING TIME:
30 minutes

CRUSTED TEMPEH STRIPS WITH ROAST BRUSSELS SPROUTS & MUSHROOM SAUCE

Tempeh, cooked well, tastes amazing when paired with great flavours.

SERVES 2

480 g (1 lb 1 oz) brussels sprouts, halved
1 pinch each salt and freshly ground black pepper
1 garlic clove, finely chopped
300 g (10½ oz) tempeh, cut into 1 cm (⅜ inch) strips
45 g (1¾ oz/¼ cup) chia seeds
40 g (1½ oz/¼ cup) black sesame seeds

MARINADE
2 tablespoons finely grated fresh ginger
1 tablespoon sesame oil
1 tablespoon tamari (gluten-free soy sauce)

MUSHROOM SAUCE
125 ml (4 fl oz/½ cup) almond milk
50 g (1¾ oz/1 cup) fresh shiitake mushrooms, finely chopped
1 tablespoon tamari
1 small kale leaf, finely chopped, stalk removed (about ½ cup)

Preheat the oven to 160°C (315°F). Spread the brussels sprouts on a lightly greased baking tray, season with the salt and pepper, toss with the garlic and roast for 15 minutes or until golden.

Meanwhile, combine all of the marinade ingredients in a bowl. Add the tempeh and stir to coat well, then set aside to marinate for 10 minutes.

To make the mushroom sauce, put the almond milk, mushrooms and tamari in a saucepan and simmer over medium heat for 10 minutes or until reduced by one-quarter. Add the kale and cook for another 1–2 minutes until wilted, then remove from the heat.

Combine the chia and sesame seeds in a bowl. Remove the tempeh from the marinade, add to the seeds and toss to coat well. Reserve the marinade and the leftover seeds. Heat a nonstick frying pan over high heat. Add the tempeh and the marinade and fry for 2 minutes on each side or until golden. Divide the brussels sprouts and tempeh between two serving plates, pour the mushroom sauce over the top and sprinkle with the leftover seeds.

MISO BARRAMUNDI WITH KALE & PERUVIAN GROUNDCHERRY BROWN RICE

This miso barramundi is one of my favourites at About Life. Barramundi is an Australian native fish and is also very clean. I love the saltiness and the sweetness together with the brown rice.

SERVES 4

440 g (15½ oz/2 cups) brown rice
4 barramundi fillets, about 200 g (7 oz) each, skin on
2 tablespoons coconut oil
1 garlic clove, finely chopped
150 g (5½ oz/¾ cup) Peruvian groundcherries (Inca berries)
2 teaspoons tamari (gluten-free soy sauce)
2 large kale leaves, thinly sliced, stalks removed (about 2 cups)
2 tablespoons toasted sesame seeds
Lemon wedges, to serve

MISO CORIANDER DRESSING
145 g (5¼ oz/½ cup) white (shiro) miso
90 g (3¼ oz/⅓ cup) tahini
2 tablespoons finely chopped coriander (cilantro) leaves

Put the rice in a saucepan with 1 litre (35 fl oz/4 cups) of water and bring to the boil over high heat. Reduce the heat to as low as possible, cover with a tight-fitting lid and cook for 45 minutes. Remove from the heat and stand, covered, for 10 minutes. Do not lift the lid during cooking.

Meanwhile, make the dressing to use as a marinade. Combine all of the dressing ingredients in a bowl. Add the fish, turn to coat and allow to marinate for 15 minutes.

Heat 1 tablespoon of the coconut oil in a large nonstick frying pan over medium-high heat. Add the fish, skin-side down, and cook without moving for 10–12 minutes. Turn over and cook for another 5 minutes or until just cooked through. The cooking time will vary depending on the thickness of the fish. Remove from the pan and rest.

Heat the remaining tablespoon of coconut oil in a separate frying pan over medium heat. Add the garlic and cook for 1–2 minutes until fragrant, then add the brown rice and stir for 2–3 minutes until heated through. Add the Peruvian groundcherries and tamari and cook for another 2 minutes, then stir in the kale, season with salt and pepper and cook for another minute or until the kale is wilted and heated through.

Sprinkle the miso barramundi with the sesame seeds and serve immediately with the warm brown rice and lemon wedges.

———————

+ **NOTE** Miso is fermented soy beans. It supports the digestive system with beneficial bacteria, and has plenty of protein and other nutrients as well.

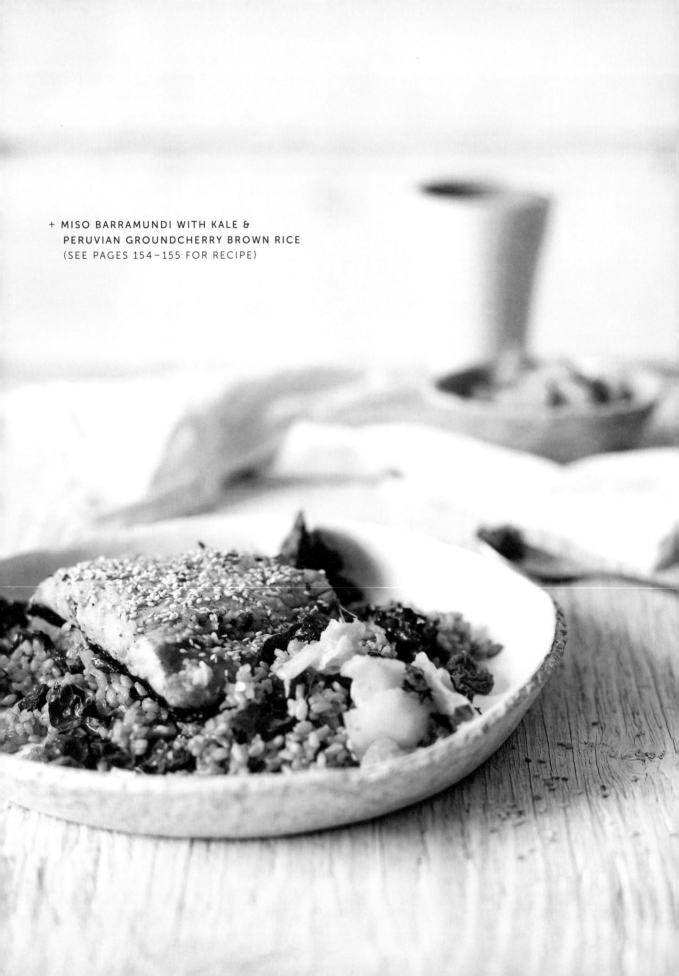

+ MISO BARRAMUNDI WITH KALE &
  PERUVIAN GROUNDCHERRY BROWN RICE
  (SEE PAGES 154–155 FOR RECIPE)

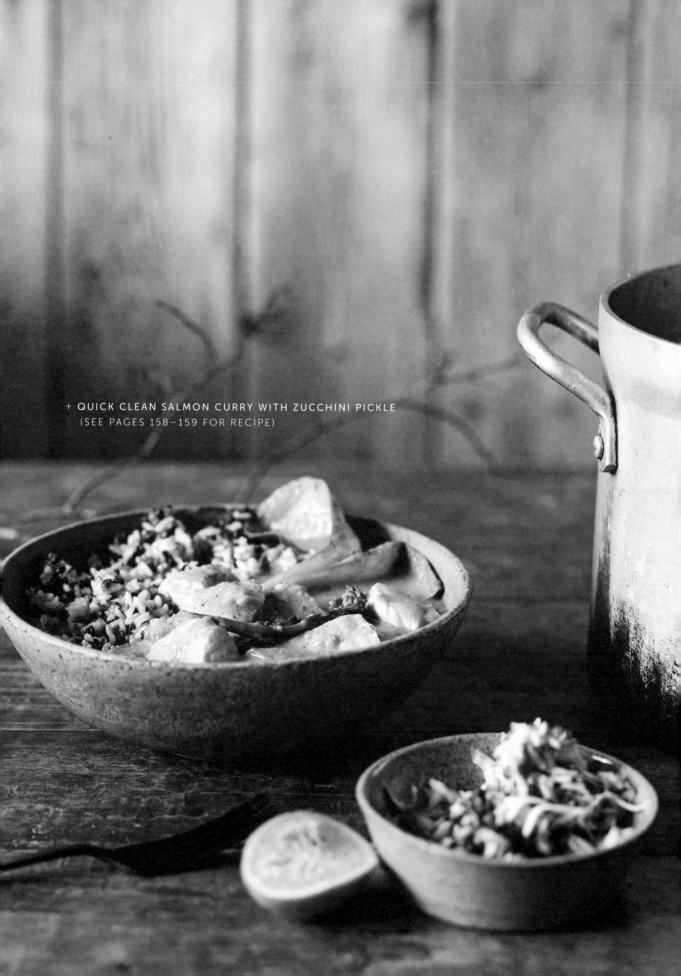

+ QUICK CLEAN SALMON CURRY WITH ZUCCHINI PICKLE
(SEE PAGES 158–159 FOR RECIPE)

QUICK CLEAN SALMON CURRY WITH ZUCCHINI PICKLE

*This recipe is such a healthy treat:
my perfect type of comfort food.*

SERVES 4

2 tablespoons coconut oil
1 onion, finely chopped
8 tomatoes, chopped
8 kaffir lime (makrut) leaves,
    thinly sliced
400 ml (14 fl oz) tin coconut milk
600 g (1 lb 5 oz) skinless salmon
    fillet, pinbones removed and
    cut into 3 cm (1¼ inch) squares
2 bunches broccolini
    (tenderstem), chopped
2 bunches bok choy (pak choy),
    chopped
65 g (2½ oz/1 cup) shredded coconut
Coriander (cilantro) leaves,
    chopped, for scattering
Lime wedges and Himalayan
    Spinach & Chia Roti
    (see page 189), to serve

ZUCCHINI PICKLE
2 zucchini (courgettes), finely
    grated
60 ml (2 fl oz/¼ cup) apple
    cider vinegar
1 teaspoon salt
15 g (½ oz/¼ cup) chopped
    coriander (cilantro) leaves

CURRY PASTE
2 garlic cloves, chopped
4 cm (1½ inch) piece fresh ginger,
    grated
3 tablespoons coriander seeds
65 g (2½ oz/¼ cup) curry powder
3 fresh long red chillies, finely
    chopped

To make the zucchini pickle, put the zucchini in a bowl with the apple cider vinegar, salt and coriander, then set aside for 20 minutes to pickle lightly. Drain and set aside.

Meanwhile, to make the curry paste, combine all of the ingredients and use a mortar and pestle or a small food processor to grind to a paste.

Heat the coconut oil in a frying pan over medium heat. Add the onion and cook for 3–4 minutes until soft. Add the curry paste and cook for 2 minutes or until fragrant. Add the tomato and kaffir lime leaves and cook for 2 minutes, then add the coconut milk and bring to a simmer for 10 minutes. Season with salt and freshly ground black pepper and stir. Add the salmon and cook for 7 minutes. Gently stir in the broccolini and bok choy, remove from the heat and stand for 1–2 minutes.

Divide the curry among four serving bowls, top with the shredded coconut and a little of the zucchini pickle, Scatter with the chopped coriander leaves, then serve with lime wedges and Himalayan roti.

———————

+ **NOTE** I like to serve this dish with Black Pearl Medley, a combination of wholegrain brown rice, black barley and daikon radish seeds. Put 400 g (14 oz/2 cups) black pearl medley in a saucepan with 1 litre (35 fl oz/4 cups) of cold water. Bring to the boil over high heat, cover and reduce heat to low, then simmer until all of the water is absorbed and the medley is soft.

PREP TIME:
30 minutes

COOKING TIME:
25 minutes

PURPLE CABBAGE DUMPLINGS WITH ALMOND BUTTER HOISIN SAUCE

Dumplings are great but often too heavy. This is a lighter version using yummy filled cabbage cups.

SERVES 4–6

1 purple cabbage
500 g (1 lb 2 oz) minced (ground)
    pork or chicken
2 spring onions (scallions),
    finely chopped
⅓ cup finely grated fresh ginger
90 g (3¼ oz/½ cup) drained water
    chestnuts, coarsely chopped
2 garlic cloves, finely chopped
1½ tablespoons tamari
    (gluten-free soy sauce)
2 tablespoons chia seeds
1 egg

ALMOND BUTTER HOISIN SAUCE
60 ml (2 fl oz/¼ cup) tamari
    (gluten-free soy sauce)
3 tablespoons almond butter
2 tablespoons raw honey
2 tablespoons tahini
2 teaspoons mirin (rice wine)
3 teaspoons sesame oil
1 garlic clove, finely chopped
½ teaspoon dried chilli flakes
1 teaspoon white (shiro) miso
1 teaspoon Cinnamon Five Spice
    (see page 174)

Peel off 16 of the outer cabbage leaves. Cook the leaves in a large saucepan of boiling water for 2 minutes, then drain and submerge in a large bowl of iced water to stop them cooking further. When cool, drain and pat dry on a large clean tea towel (dish towel). Using a small sharp knife, trim the thick ribs from the end of the leaves: this will make them easier to roll.

Finely chop 100 g (3½ oz) of the remaining cabbage and put it in a bowl with the remaining ingredients. Mix well to combine. Divide the mixture into 16 portions and place one in each cabbage leaf.

Working with one at a time, roll up the cabbage leaf around the filling, folding in the sides as you go, and secure with toothpicks. Place the dumpling seam-side down in the top of a steamer basket. Repeat with the remaining cabbage leaves and filling to make 16 dumplings. Steam for 15–20 minutes or until the meat is well cooked.

Meanwhile, to make the dipping sauce, combine all of the ingredients in a bowl and stir to mix well.

Serve the hot dumplings and the remaining balls with the dipping sauce on the side.

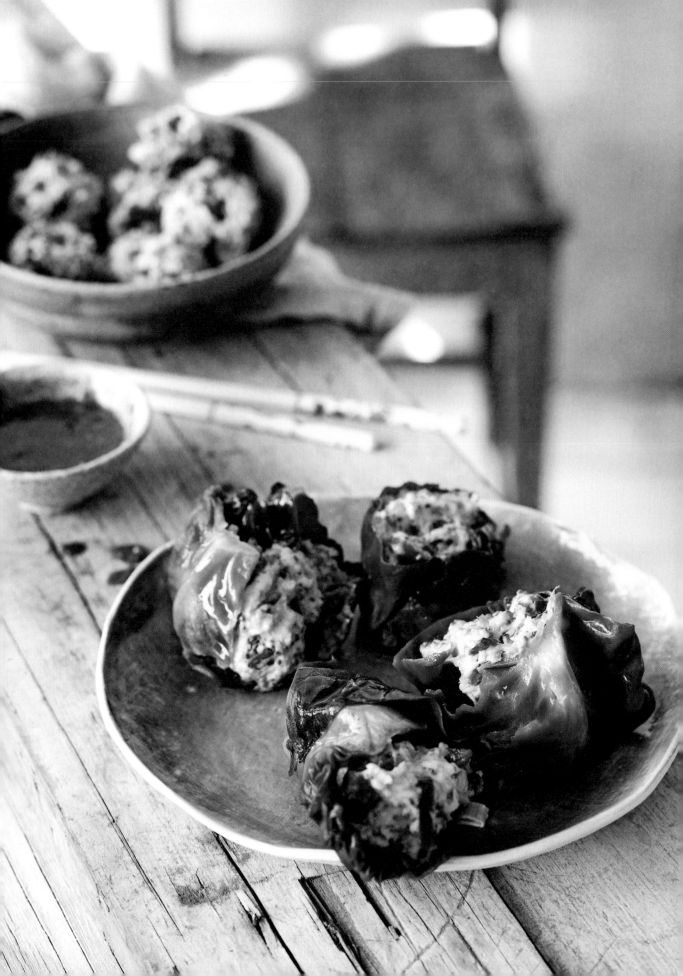

PREP TIME:
*25 minutes,
plus 20 minutes
standing time*

COOKING TIME:
50 minutes

MACADAMIA BUTTER CHICKEN

I love butter chicken, but it always seems very intimidating to make. This recipe is quite an easy one and full of flavour.

SERVES 4

800 g (1 lb 12 oz) skinless chicken thigh fillets, cut into thirds
90 g (3¼ oz/2 cups) baby spinach leaves
1 teaspoon chopped coriander (cilantro) leaves
Cauliflower & Broccoli Mash (see page 193) and Greek-style yoghurt, to serve

MARINADE
130 g (4½ oz/½ cup) Greek-style yoghurt
80 ml (2½ fl oz/⅓ cup) olive oil
2 teaspoons lemon juice
1 teaspoon finely grated garlic
1 teaspoon finely grated ginger
1 teaspoon dried chilli flakes
1 teaspoon garam masala
1 teaspoon ground turmeric
1 teaspoon ground cumin

SAUCE
60 ml (2 fl oz/¼ cup) olive oil
2 tablespoons finely grated garlic
2 teaspoons finely grated ginger
2 teaspoons dried chilli flakes
1 teaspoon garam masala
1 teaspoon ground turmeric
1 teaspoon ground cardamom
1 teaspoon ground coriander
½ teaspoon ground cloves
400 g (14 oz) tin chopped tomatoes
80 ml (2½ fl oz/⅓ cup) lemon juice
250 ml (9 fl oz/1 cup) coconut cream
2 teaspoons ghee
1 teaspoon salt
120 g (4¼ oz/1 cup) coarsely chopped macadamia nuts

Preheat the oven to 180°C (350°F).

To make the marinade, put all of the ingredients into a large mixing bowl and stir to combine well. Add the chicken, toss to coat well and marinate in the fridge for 20 minutes. Transfer the marinated chicken to a baking tray and roast for 20 minutes or until just cooked through.

To make the sauce, heat a saucepan over medium-high heat. Add the olive oil, garlic, ginger and spices and stir for 2 minutes or until fragrant. Add the chopped tomatoes, reduce the heat to low and cook, stirring occasionally, for 10 minutes or until slightly thickened and reduced. Add the chicken along with any cooking juices, then stir in the lemon juice and cook for another 5 minutes. Add the coconut cream and ghee and simmer for 10 minutes or until reduced and thickened. Add the salt, then stir in the chopped macadamias. Remove from the heat and stir through the spinach and coriander.

Serve with the broccoli and cauliflower mash and yoghurt.

+ **NOTE** Ghee is a nutritious, lactose-free form of butter and is great for digestive health and boosting immunity.

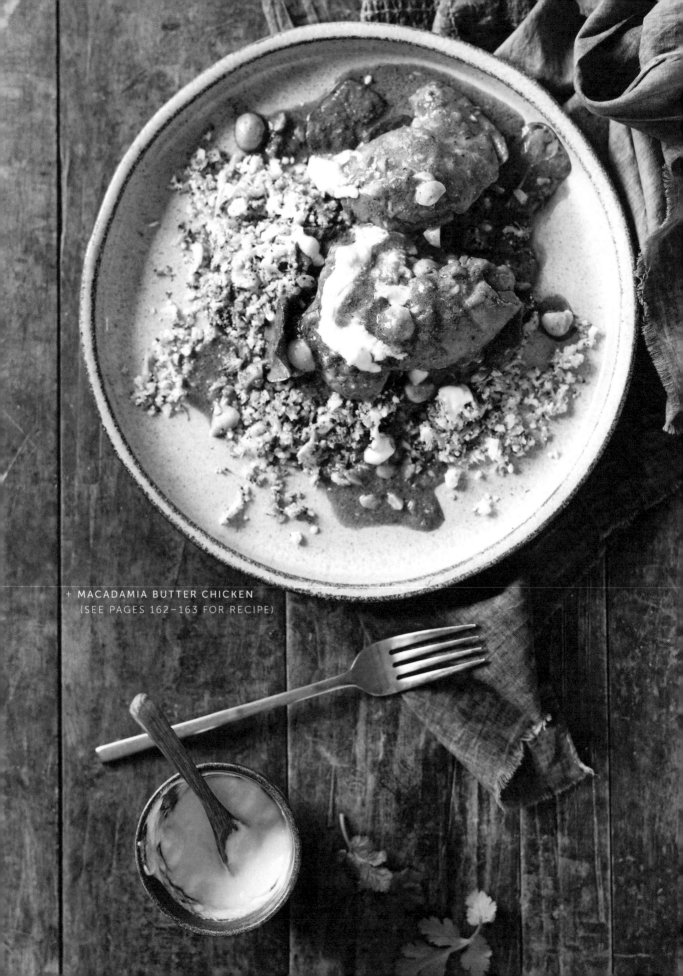

+ MACADAMIA BUTTER CHICKEN
(SEE PAGES 162–163 FOR RECIPE)

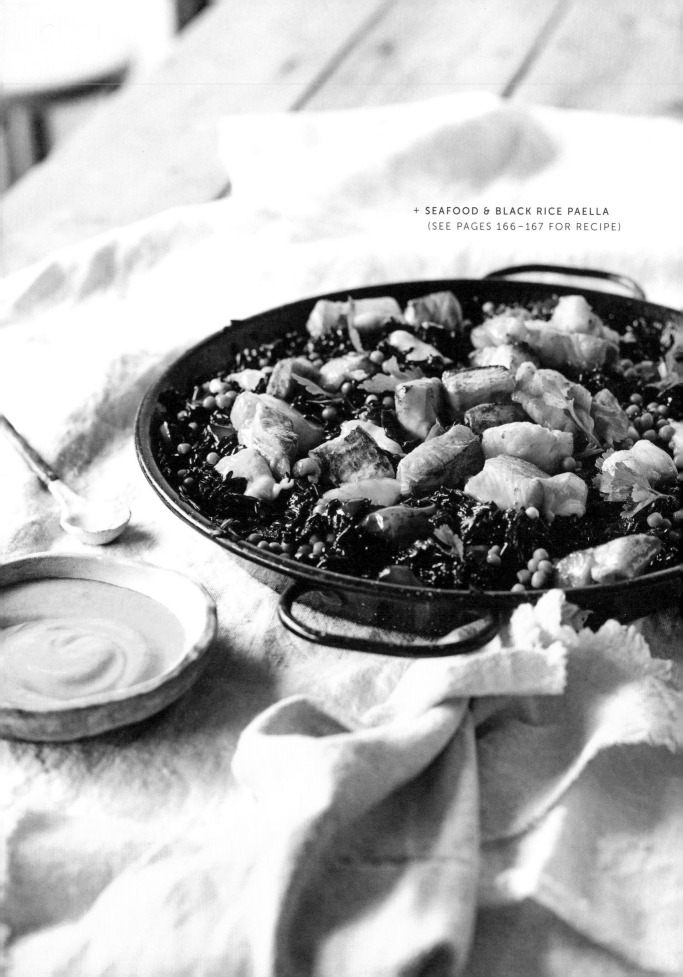

+ SEAFOOD & BLACK RICE PAELLA
(SEE PAGES 166–167 FOR RECIPE)

SEAFOOD & BLACK RICE PAELLA

Treat your loved one to a romantic and nutritious dinner with this flavour-loaded seafood and black rice paella. This version is fish only, but feel free to add other seafood such as prawns (shrimp) and mussels. If you prefer, you can substitute chicken and chorizo for the fish.

SERVES 4

2 tablespoons ghee
1 onion, finely chopped
2 garlic cloves, finely chopped
2 red capsicums (peppers), seeds and membranes removed, thinly sliced
600 g (1 lb 5 oz/3 cups) black rice
1 teaspoon ground turmeric
2 teaspoons smoked paprika
4 tomatoes, chopped
250 ml (9 fl oz/1 cup) white wine
2 teaspoons dried mixed herbs
2 teaspoons dried chilli flakes
1.5 litres (52 fl oz/6 cups) Bone Broth (see page 99) or Nourishing Vegie & Potato Broth (see page 95)
400 g (14 oz) skinless salmon fillet, pinbones removed, cut into 3 cm (1¼ inch) pieces

400 g (14 oz) skinless firm white-fleshed fish fillets, cut into 3 cm (1¼ inch) pieces
280 g (10 oz/2 cups) frozen peas
90 g (3¼ oz/1½ cups) coarsely chopped parsley
Lime wedges, to serve

TURMERIC AÏOLI
135 g (4¾ oz/½ cup) tahini
Juice of ½ lemon
1 teaspoon salt
60 ml (2 fl oz/¼ cup) olive oil
2 teaspoons ground turmeric
1 garlic clove, minced

Preheat the oven to 180°C (350°F).

Melt 1 tablespoon of the ghee in a paella pan or large ovenproof frying pan over medium heat. Add the onion and cook gently for 5 minutes or until soft but not coloured. Add the garlic and capsicum and stir for 2–3 minutes, then add the rice, turmeric and 1½ teaspoons of the paprika and stir well. Add the tomato and stir for a few minutes or until the rice is well coated and lightly toasted. Stir in the wine and cook for 1–2 minutes to allow the alcohol to burn off, then stir in the mixed herbs and chilli flakes. Add a couple of ladles of broth, reduce the heat to low and stir until all the liquid is absorbed. Continue adding broth, one ladle at a time, allowing each addition to be absorbed before adding the next.

Meanwhile, melt the remaining ghee in a frying pan over medium heat. Add the remaining ½ teaspoon of paprika and stir for 1 minute. Increase the heat to medium-high, add the salmon and white fish and cook for 1–2 minutes until brown on both sides. Remove the fish from the pan. If you want to add extra seafood, add it to the pan at this point and fry it for 1–2 minutes until lightly coloured.

Place the fish pieces on top of the rice, nestling the fish into the rice a little. Transfer the pan to the oven and bake for 10 minutes. Add more broth if it is needed and stir the rice gently, making sure you do not break up the fish. Add the peas and cook for another 5–10 minutes until the rice and seafood are cooked.

To make the turmeric aïoli, combine all of the ingredients in a small bowl. Add 60 ml (2 fl oz/¼ cup) of water and use a fork to combine well. Serve the paella scattered with the chopped parsley and lime wedges, and serve the turmeric aïoli on the side.

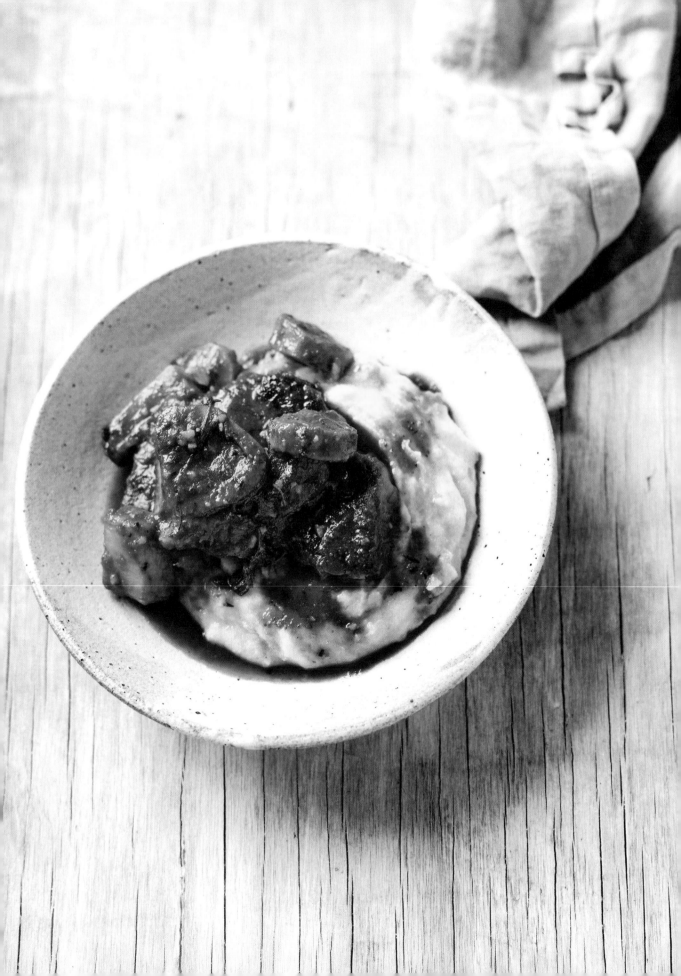

+ GLUTEN-FREE
+ DAIRY-FREE
+ PALEO

PREP TIME:
20 minutes, plus overnight marinating

COOKING TIME:
8¼ hours

CHAI-SPICED OSSO BUCCO IN THE SLOW COOKER

This is a great recipe to throw together before you head out the door so that you come home to a delicious dinner ready to go: yum!

SERVES 4

800 g (1 lb 12 oz) osso bucco
    (veal shin, bone in)
2 garlic cloves, finely chopped
500 ml (17 fl oz/2 cups) freshly
    brewed black chai tea, cooled
60 ml (2 fl oz/¼ cup) olive oil
2 tablespoons ghee
500 ml (17 fl oz/2 cups) red wine
3 carrots, chopped
3 purple carrots, chopped
2 onions, quartered
20 g (¾ oz/about 10) dried
    porcini mushrooms
500 ml (17 fl oz/2 cups) tomato
    passata (puréed tomatoes)
1 bunch thyme, leaves chopped
250 ml (9 fl oz/1 cup) Bone Broth
    (see page 99)

CREAMY MISO POLENTA
190 g (6¾ oz/1 cup) polenta
50 g (1 ¾ oz) ghee
1 tablespoon thyme leaves, chopped
3 tablespoons white (shiro) miso

Combine the osso bucco, garlic, tea and olive oil in a large airtight container and refrigerate overnight.

Drain the osso bucco, reserving the liquid, and pat the meat dry with paper towel. Heat the ghee in a large frying pan over high heat. Cook the osso bucco until golden on both sides, then transfer to a slow cooker. Deglaze the frying pan with the wine and add to the slow cooker. Add the remaining ingredients and reserved marinating liquid. Season with salt and freshly ground black pepper and cook on Low for 8 hours or until the meat is falling off the bone.

Just before serving, bring 1 litre (35 fl oz/4 cups) of water to the boil in a saucepan. Whisking constantly, gradually add the polenta and season with salt. Reduce heat to low and continue to whisk for 5 minutes, then add the ghee, thyme and miso. Stir over low heat for a further 3 minutes or until thick and creamy.

Serve the osso bucco on a bed of polenta and enjoy this nourishing bowl of goodness with a glass of red wine.

+ **NOTE** Don't have a slow cooker? You can cook this in the oven at 160°C (315°F) for 2 hours or until tender.

SIDES

+ VEGETARIAN
+ VEGAN
+ GLUTEN-FREE
+ DAIRY-FREE
+ PALEO
+ RAW

PREP TIME:
*15 minutes, plus
2 days pickling*

COOKING TIME:
Nil

PICKLED KIMCHI

Spicy and easy to make, pickled cabbage is a great addition to any meal. In this recipe the Peruvian groundcherries (Inca berries) have an amazing flavour that pops in your mouth.

MAKES 3½ CUPS

3 cups sliced Chinese cabbage
    (wong bok)
1 small kale leaf, thinly sliced,
    stalks removed (about ½ cup)
½ cup Peruvian groundcherries
    (Inca berries)
2 tablespoons grated fresh ginger
2 tablespoons raw sugar
2 tablespoons apple cider vinegar
2 teaspoons pink Himalayan salt
1 garlic clove, finely chopped
½ teaspoon cayenne pepper
1 pinch dried chilli flakes

Put all of the ingredients in a large bowl with 375 ml (13 fl oz/1½ cups) of water and combine well. Transfer to a large jar and press the contents down tightly. If necessary, add a little extra water to cover the vegetables, ensuring they are submerged completely. Seal and refrigerate for 2 days before serving.

+ **NOTE** Pickling is a form of fermentation and helps to break down the hard-to-digest cellulose in the vegies. As a Slovakian, I am very used to having pickled vegies with every meal to help digestion. Reduce waste by pickling leftover vegies to preserve both the food and the environment.

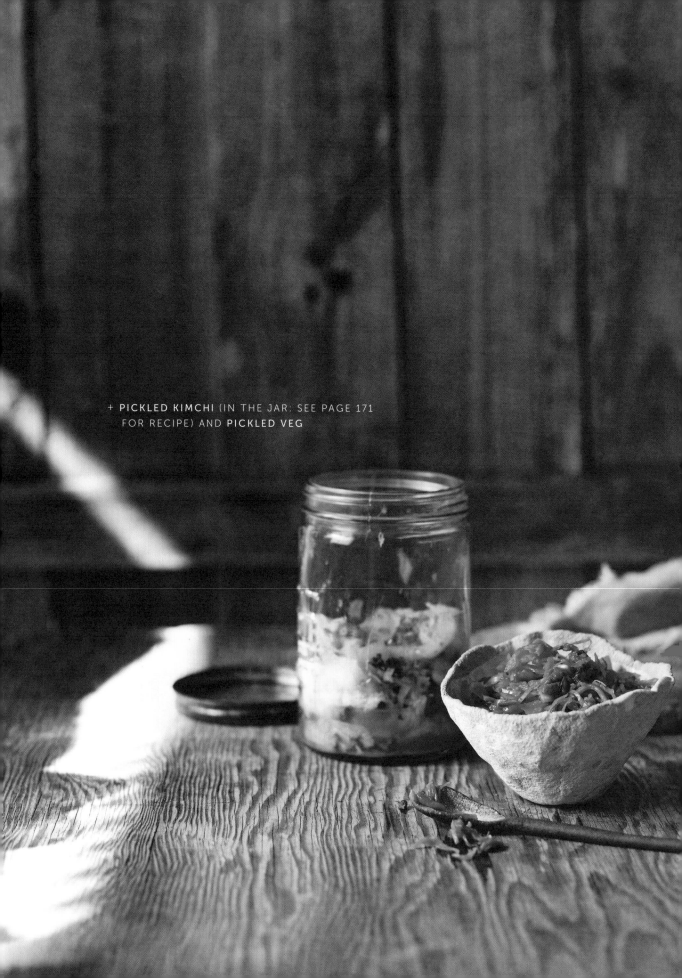

+ **PICKLED KIMCHI** (IN THE JAR: SEE PAGE 171 FOR RECIPE) AND **PICKLED VEG**

+ VEGETARIAN
+ VEGAN
+ GLUTEN-FREE
+ DAIRY-FREE
+ RAW

PREP TIME:
*15 minutes, plus
2 days pickling*

COOKING TIME:
Nil

PICKLED VEG

*This amazing hot pink pickle adds colour
and flavour to any meal.*

MAKES ABOUT 2½ CUPS

*100 g (3½ oz) purple cabbage,
    shredded*
*100 g (3½ oz) white cabbage,
    shredded*
*1 kale leaf, thinly sliced, stalk
    discarded (about 1 cup)*
30 g (1 oz/¼ cup) goji berries
*2 tablespoons raw honey,
    or use vegan sweetener*
2 teaspoons pink Himalayan salt
2 tablespoons apple cider vinegar
¼ teaspoon coriander seeds
¼ teaspoon cumin seeds
¼ teaspoon fennel seeds
1 tablespoon lemon juice

Put all of the ingredients in a large bowl with 375 ml (13 fl oz/1½ cups) of water and combine well. Transfer to a large jar or airtight container and press the cabbage down firmly to compact. If necessary, add a little extra water to cover the cabbage, ensuring it is submerged in liquid. Seal and refrigerate for 2 days before serving.

+ **NOTE** Goji berries are laced with vitamins, minerals and have a very high protein and fibre content. They are great to eat as a snack or add to breakfast cereals and salads.

THREE HEALING
SPICE BLENDS

+ VEGETARIAN
+ VEGAN
+ GLUTEN-FREE
+ DAIRY-FREE
+ PALEO

PREP TIME:
5 minutes

COOKING TIME:
Nil

CINNAMON
FIVE SPICE

*Use this in smoothies and hot drinks,
or as a spicy rub for meat or fish.*

MAKES ⅔ CUP

4 tablespoons ground cinnamon
1 tablespoon ground fennel
1¼ tablespoons ground star anise
3 teaspoons ground black pepper
1 teaspoon ground cloves
1 teaspoon pink Himalayan salt

Put all of the ingredients in a small jar
or airtight container, seal and shake to
combine. The mixture will keep in a cool
dark place for up to 1 month.

+ **NOTE** Cinnamon is a blood sugar
regulator. I love this spice and I sprinkle it
on my coffee every day: being creative in
the kitchen really should have no limits.

+ VEGETARIAN
+ VEGAN
+ GLUTEN-FREE
+ DAIRY-FREE
+ PALEO

PREP TIME:
5 minutes

COOKING TIME:
Nil

DIGESTIVE SPICE

Perfect for curries, dressings and with grain-based dishes.

MAKES ⅔ CUP

4 tablespoons ground turmeric
1½ tablespoons ground cinnamon
1½ tablespoons ground ginger
1 tablespoon ground fennel

Put all of the ingredients in a small jar or airtight container, seal and shake to combine. The mixture will keep in a cool dark place for up to 1 month.

+ **NOTE** Ginger and fennel are powerful digestive herbs. I use this spice mix in my salad dressings.

+ VEGETARIAN
+ VEGAN
+ GLUTEN-FREE
+ DAIRY-FREE
+ PALEO

PREP TIME:
5 minutes

COOKING TIME:
Nil

BEAT SUGAR CRAVINGS

This mix is great in smoothies and hot drinks, or sprinkled on yoghurt.

MAKES ⅔ CUP

4 tablespoons ground cinnamon
1½ tablespoons ground ginger
1½ tablespoons ground cloves
1 tablespoon ground nutmeg

Put all of the ingredients in a small jar or airtight container, seal and shake to combine. The mixture will keep in a cool dark place for up to 1 month.

+ **NOTE** Nutmeg has antimicrobial and anti-inflammatory properties, as well as a delicious sweet flavour.

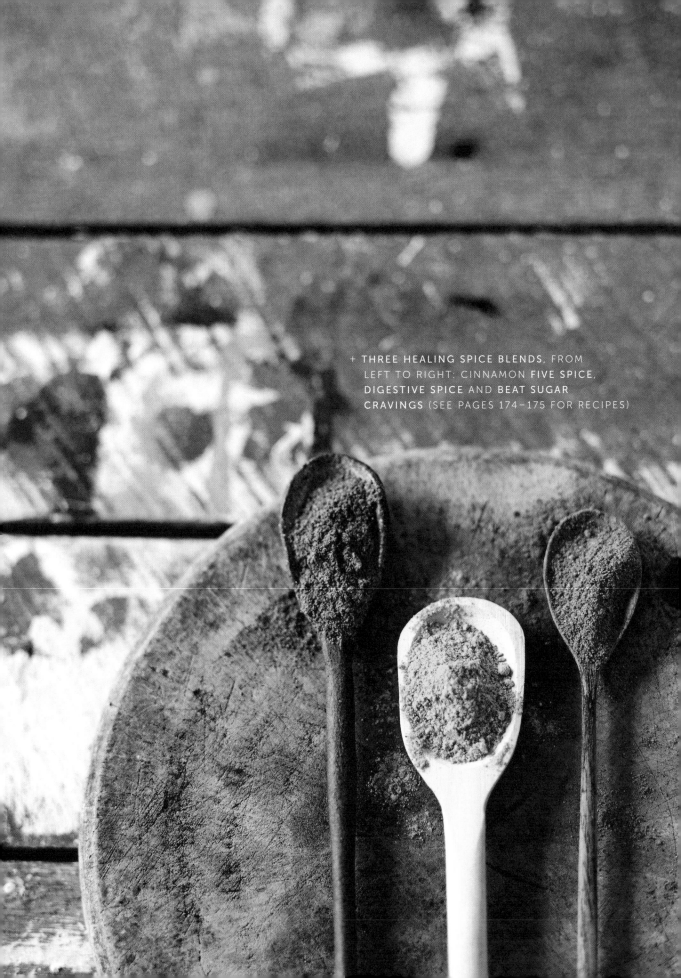

+ THREE HEALING SPICE BLENDS, FROM LEFT TO RIGHT: CINNAMON FIVE SPICE, DIGESTIVE SPICE AND BEAT SUGAR CRAVINGS (SEE PAGES 174–175 FOR RECIPES)

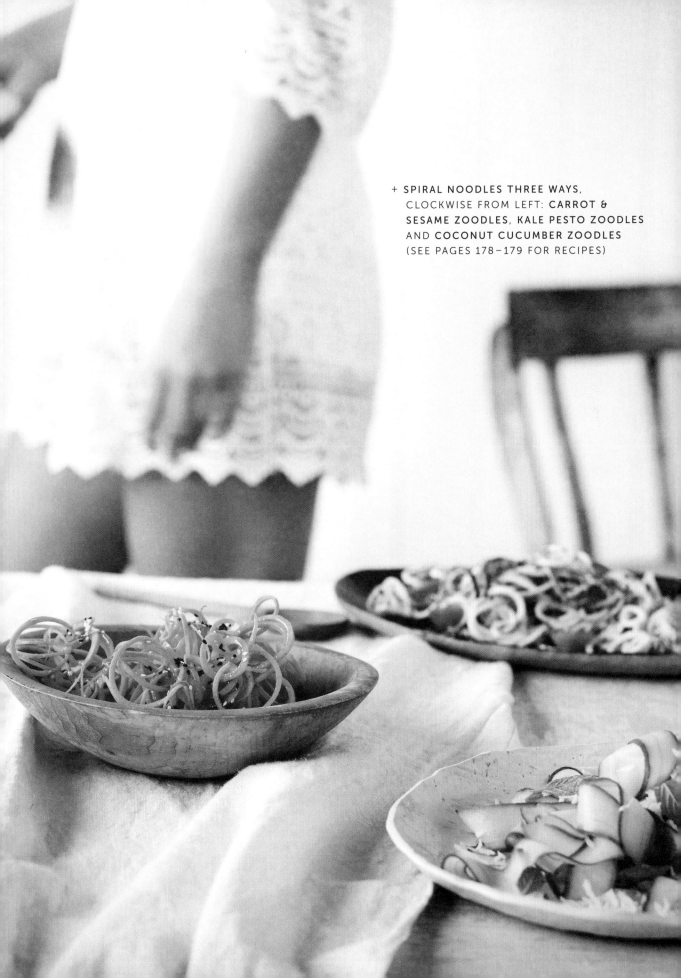

+ SPIRAL NOODLES THREE WAYS,
CLOCKWISE FROM LEFT: **CARROT &
SESAME ZOODLES, KALE PESTO ZOODLES**
AND **COCONUT CUCUMBER ZOODLES**
(SEE PAGES 178–179 FOR RECIPES)

SPIRAL NOODLES
THREE WAYS

+ VEGETARIAN
+ VEGAN
+ GLUTEN-FREE
+ DAIRY-FREE
+ PALEO
+ RAW

PREP TIME:
10 minutes

COOKING TIME:
Nil

KALE PESTO
ZOODLES

Fresh, zingy and great to pair with Quinoa Meatballs (see page 139).

SERVES 4

3 large zucchini (courgettes), ends trimmed
4 tablespoons Activated Raw Kale Pesto
   (see page 60)
2 tablespoons lemon juice
170 g (6 oz) cherry tomatoes, halved
2 tablespoons linseeds (flaxseeds)

Using a spiraliser, cut the zucchini into noodles. Alternatively, use a vegetable peeler to slice the zucchini lengthways into long thin ribbons; it will look more like fettuccine but will be just as delicious.

Put the zucchini in a large bowl, add the remaining ingredients and toss to combine well. Transfer to a serving bowl and serve immediately.

+ **NOTE** Zucchini noodles are a good substitute for pasta.

+ VEGETARIAN
+ VEGAN
+ GLUTEN-FREE
+ DAIRY-FREE
+ PALEO
+ RAW

PREP TIME:
10 minutes

COOKING TIME:
Nil

CARROT & SESAME ZOODLES

Try these vegie spirals with Miso Barramundi with Kale (see page 154).

SERVES 4

3 large carrots, washed, tops removed
1½ tablespoons sesame oil
2 tablespoons tamari (gluten-free soy sauce)
2 tablespoons white sesame seeds
2 tablespoons black sesame seeds

Using a spiraliser, cut the carrots into noodles. Alternatively, use a vegetable peeler to slice the carrots lengthways into long thin ribbons; it will look more like fettuccine but will be just as delicious.

Put the carrot in a large bowl, add the remaining ingredients and toss to combine well. Transfer to a serving bowl and serve immediately.

+ **NOTE** Carrots are power vegetables with loads of fibre and betacarotene.

+ VEGETARIAN
+ VEGAN
+ GLUTEN-FREE
+ DAIRY-FREE
+ PALEO
+ RAW

PREP TIME:
10 minutes

COOKING TIME:
Nil

COCONUT CUCUMBER ZOODLES

This is a perfect accompaniment for Turmeric & Lime Coconut Baked Snapper (see page 128).

SERVES 4

3 Lebanese (short) cucumbers
2 tablespoons lime juice
20 g (¾ oz/½ cup) coconut chips
10 g (⅜ oz/⅓ cup) torn mint leaves
¼ teaspoon salt

Using a spiraliser, cut the cucumbers into noodles. Alternatively, use a vegetable peeler to slice the cucumbers lengthways into long thin ribbons: it will look more like fettuccine but will be just as delicious.

Put the cucumber in a large bowl, add the remaining ingredients and toss to combine well. Transfer to a serving bowl and serve immediately.

+ **NOTE** Cucumber's high water content makes it a great detox food.

KALE & LINSEED SPANAKOPITA

*I love spanakopita, and this is a beautiful twist
on the traditional recipe, using high-quality
ingredients. It is a dish meant for sharing,
so it's great for entertaining.*

SERVES 4–6

1 sheet ready-rolled puff pastry
*100 g (3½ oz/1 cup) grated
    pecorino cheese*
*100 g (3½ oz/1 cup) crumbled
    feta cheese*
*15 g (½ oz/½ cup) chopped
    flat-leaf (Italian) parsley*
*4 kale leaves, thinly sliced, stalks
    removed (about 4 cups)*
3 garlic cloves, finely chopped
*1 tablespoon chopped thyme
    leaves*
4 tablespoons linseeds (flaxseeds)
*65 g (2½ oz/⅓ cup) Peruvian
    groundcherries (Inca berries)*
55 g (2 oz/⅓ cup) quark
1 egg yolk, lightly beaten

Preheat the oven to 180°C (350°F). Line a baking tray
with baking paper and lay the sheet of pastry on it.

Put all of the remaining ingredients, except the egg yolk,
in a mixing bowl and stir until well combined. Spread
the mixture evenly over the top of the pastry, leaving
a 1 cm (⅜ inch) border, then roll up into a tight roll.
Refrigerate, seam-side down, on the tray for 15 minutes.

Using a large sharp knife, cut the roll in half lengthways.
Form a ring with each half with the cut (open) side
up. Brush all over with the beaten egg yolk. Bake for
40 minutes or until golden and crisp. Serve warm or
at room temperature.

+ **NOTE** Quark is a German-style cottage cheese that
    can be used as a substitute for sour cream. It is often
    used in cheesecakes.

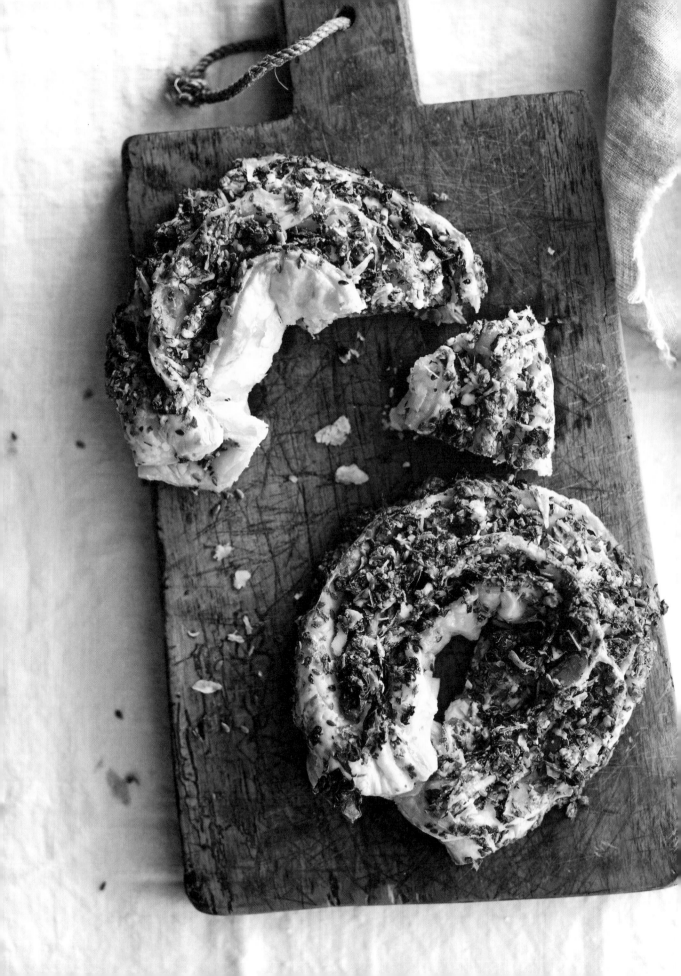

PREP TIME:
15 minutes

COOKING TIME:
10 minutes

GARAM MASALA CREAMED SPINACH

This spinach-based side dish can be used as a companion to any meal, especially crusted tofu, chicken or even a fried egg. My mum used to make a quick dinner of creamed spinach with an egg on top. Just as it did for Popeye, spinach helps you grow muscles and gives you green power! Here is my mum's version with a twist.

SERVES 4

1 teaspoon fennel seeds
1 tablespoon coconut oil
2 tablespoons finely chopped garlic
120 g (4¼ oz/1 cup) finely chopped spring onions (scallions)
4 large kale leaves, coarsely chopped, stalks removed (about 4 cups)
360 g (12¾ oz/8 cups) baby spinach leaves
500 ml (17 fl oz/2 cups) tinned coconut milk
½ teaspoon salt
1 teaspoon garam masala
½ teaspoon cayenne pepper

Put the fennel seeds in a dry frying pan and shake over low heat for 2–3 minutes until fragrant. Transfer to a small bowl and set aside.

Return the pan to low to medium heat. Add the coconut oil, then the garlic and stir for 2 minutes or until golden. Add the spring onion and cook for 1 minute or until soft. Stir in the kale and 135 g (4¾ oz/3 cups) of the spinach until just wilted. Add the coconut milk and the salt, bring to a simmer and cook for 2 minutes. Stir in the garam masala, cayenne pepper and fennel seeds, then remove from the heat. Stir through the remaining spinach until wilted, then check the seasoning and serve.

+ **NOTE** Dark green spinach is nutrient dense, and is a good source of vegetable iron. Add a squeeze of lemon so that the vitamin C will help you absorb the iron.

+ VEGETARIAN
+ VEGAN
+ GLUTEN-FREE
+ DAIRY-FREE
+ PALEO

PREP TIME:
5 minutes

COOKING TIME:
5 minutes

WILTED BEET TOPS WITH WARRIGAL GREENS

My favourite thing is to really use the whole vegetable, including the leaves from celery, beetroot tops and the stems and roots of herbs. This dish is perfect served with poached eggs and feta for brekkie or lunch.

SERVES 4

300 g (10½ oz) warrigal greens,
    rinsed and chopped
2 bunches beetroot (beet) leaves,
    rinsed well and chopped
80 ml (2½ fl oz/⅓ cup) olive oil
2 garlic cloves, finely chopped
Juice of 1 lemon
½ teaspoon each salt and freshly
    ground black pepper
Extra virgin olive oil, for drizzling

Rinse the greens and leaves well, then coarsely chop.

Heat the olive oil in a large frying pan over medium heat. Add the garlic and stir for 1–2 minutes until light golden. Add the greens and leaves and toss for 5–7 minutes until wilted and tender, then add the lemon juice, salt and pepper. Serve immediately drizzled with a little extra virgin olive oil.

+ **NOTE** Warrigal greens are a delicious native Australian bush food. If you can't find them, use baby spinach leaves instead.

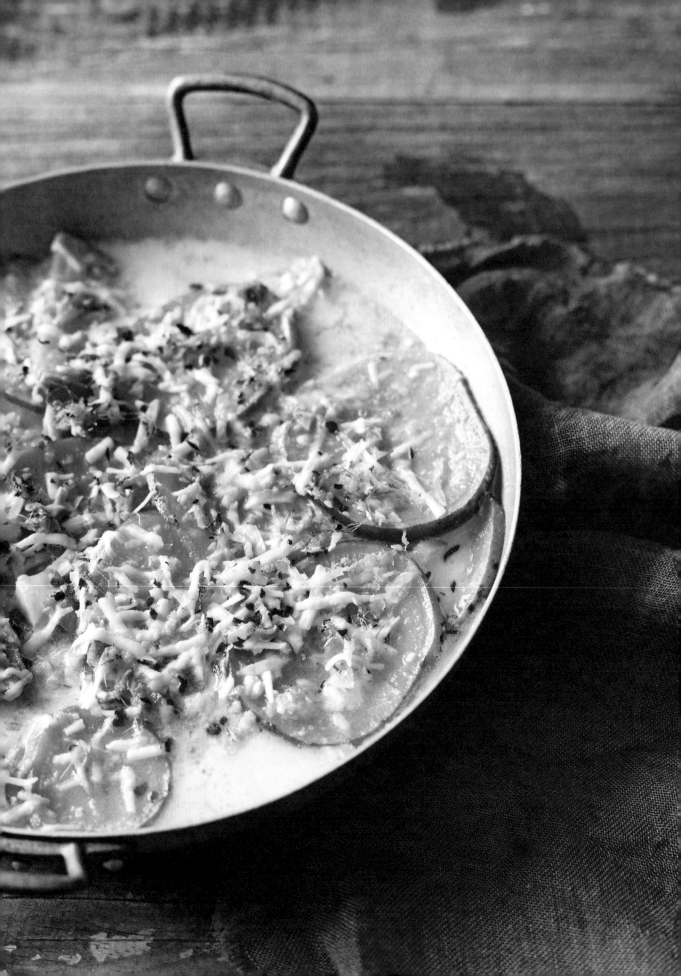

+ VEGETARIAN
+ GLUTEN-FREE
+ PALEO

PREP TIME:
20 minutes

COOKING TIME:
50 minutes

COCONUT CHILLI GINGER SWEET POTATO GRATIN

This recipe was invented by turning a classic dish on its head and using sweet potatoes instead of regular white potatoes. The chilli and ginger give it a lovely twist, too.

SERVES 4

2 large sweet potatoes (about 900 g/2 lb), washed
1 tablespoon chopped thyme leaves
1 teaspoon finely chopped garlic
375 ml (13 fl oz/1½ cups) tinned coconut milk
260 g (9¼ oz/1 cup) Greek-style yoghurt or goat's milk yoghurt
½ teaspoon salt
¼ cup finely grated fresh ginger
100 g (3½ oz/1 cup) grated parmesan cheese
½ teaspoon dried chilli flakes

Preheat the oven to 180°C (350°F).

Slice the sweet potato into thin rounds about 5 mm (¼ inch) thick, leaving the skin on. Put the slices into a saucepan with the thyme, garlic, coconut milk, yoghurt and salt and cook over medium heat, stirring occasionally, for 20 minutes or until just tender. Transfer to a shallow baking dish (about 1.5 litre/52 fl oz/6 cup capacity), cover with foil and bake for 20 minutes.

Combine the ginger and parmesan in a small bowl. After 20 minutes of cooking, remove the foil from the sweet potatoes, scatter with the ginger mixture, then sprinkle with the chilli flakes. Bake for another 10 minutes or until golden. Serve immediately.

+ **NOTE** The orangey colour of sweet potato shows that it is high in carotenoids. I love the way that nature gives us the clues about the benefits we can get from fresh produce. This dish has fat, not just for taste purposes, but also to help increase the absorption of some of the nutrients such as betacarotene.

+ VEGETARIAN
+ GLUTEN-FREE

PREP TIME:
25 minutes

COOKING TIME:
1 hour

THYME & FETA PISTACHIO LOAF

I like to experiment with new flavours and this loaf is both sweet and salty. It's lovely to eat on its own or as an afternoon-tea cake, and it is equally delicious warm or cold.

SERVES 6 (MAKES 1 LOAF)

4 eggs
75 g (2¾ oz/½ cup) rapadura
  (unrefined cane sugar)
200 g (7 oz) zucchini (courgette),
  ends trimmed, grated
130 g (4½ oz/1 cup) buckwheat
  flour
100 g (3½ oz/1 cup) almond meal
150 g (5½ oz) feta cheese, crumbled
125 ml (4 fl oz/½ cup) sweet
  almond oil
1 tablespoon thyme leaves
2 tablespoons chia seeds
2 teaspoons oregano leaves
1 teaspoon baking powder
1 pinch salt
75 g (2¾ oz/½ cup) pistachios,
  coarsely chopped

TOPPING
1 tablespoon raw honey
1 teaspoon thyme leaves
75 g (2¾ oz/½ cup) pistachios,
  coarsely chopped
65 g (2½ oz) feta cheese, crumbled

Preheat the oven to 180°C (350°F). Lightly grease a 30 x 12 x 10 cm (12 x 4½ x 4 inch) loaf (bar) tin and line the base and sides with baking paper.

Put the eggs and sugar in a mixing bowl and whisk until light and fluffy.

Put all of the remaining ingredients in a large bowl and stir to combine well. Fold in the egg mixture until well combined. Pour into the prepared tin and bake for 1 hour or until a skewer inserted into the centre comes out clean. Allow to cool in the tin for 10 minutes, then turn out onto a wire rack to cool a little more.

To serve, drizzle the loaf with the honey, then scatter with the thyme, pistachios and crumbled feta.

+ **NOTE** Buckwheat flour is a useful substitute for regular flour: it is gluten-free and it has a nutty flavour.

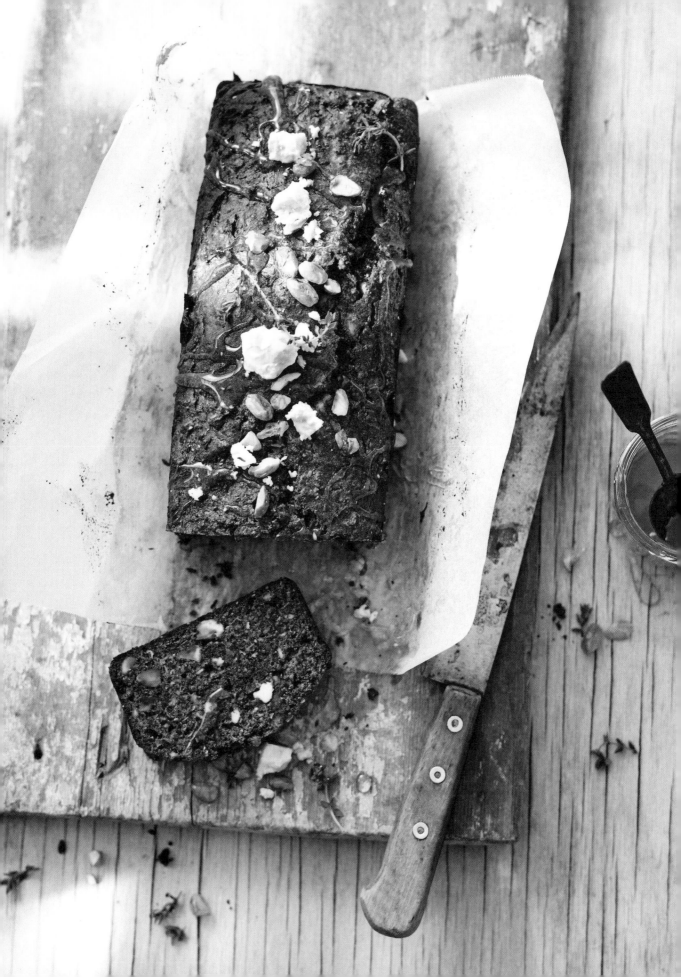

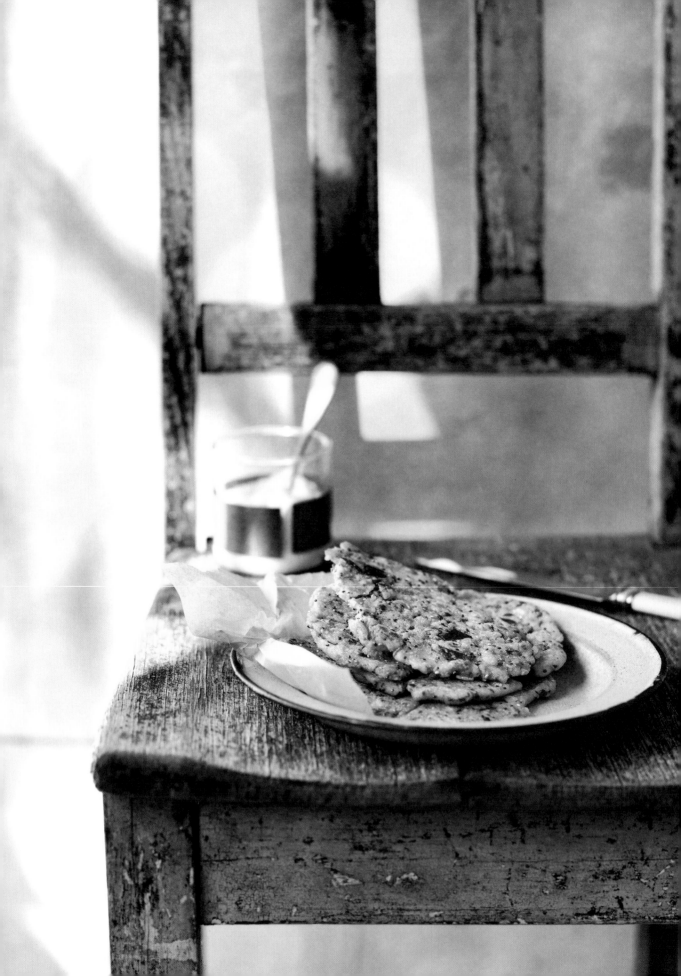

+ VEGETARIAN
+ VEGAN
+ GLUTEN-FREE
+ DAIRY-FREE

PREP TIME:
20 minutes, plus
10 minutes standing

COOKING TIME:
30 minutes

HIMALAYAN SPINACH & CHIA ROTI

*I had the inspiration for this nutritious green
bread on my travels to Mount Everest: I have
added spinach and chia. This is such a simple
recipe and good as an accompaniment to any dish,
but it is great as a breakfast bread. Just add some
eggs: the greens are already in the bread!*

MAKES 6

45 g (1½ oz/1 cup) baby spinach
    leaves
60 ml (2 fl oz/¼ cup) olive oil,
    plus extra for greasing
2 teaspoons chia seeds
½ teaspoon pink Himalayan salt
160 g (5¾ oz/1 cup) brown rice
    flour

Put the spinach and olive oil into a high-speed blender
and process until smooth. Transfer to a mixing bowl and
stir in the chia seeds and ¼ teaspoon of the salt.

Put 250 ml (9 fl oz/1 cup) of water and the remaining
¼ teaspoon of salt in a saucepan and bring to the boil.
Add the flour and stir until well combined. Remove
from the heat, cover the pan and stand for 10 minutes.
Add the flour mixture to the spinach mixture and
combine until a dough forms.

Preheat a heavy-based nonstick frying pan over medium
heat. Divide the dough into 6 pieces. Using a rolling pin
or your hands, flatten each piece into a round about
2.5 mm (⅟₁₆ inch) thick. Lightly grease the pan with oil,
then cook each roti for 2 minutes on each side or until
lightly coloured.

+ **NOTE** Roti is a crisp flat bread that is nice to serve
    as a side with curry dishes.

RYE FIVE-SPICE CARAWAY BREAD

I remember my mamička coming back from the baker with rye bread. The bread would be still warm and sometimes that's all we needed for dinner.

SERVES 6–8 (MAKES 1 LOAF)

250 ml (9 fl oz/1 cup) warm water
1½ tablespoons raw honey
2 teaspoons dry yeast
260 g (9¼ oz) rye flour
160 g (5¾ oz) spelt flour
1 teaspoon Celtic sea salt
*1 tablespoon Cinnamon Five
    Spice (see page 174)*
*1 tablespoon caraway seeds, plus
    extra for sprinkling*
60 ml (2 fl oz/¼ cup) olive oil

Combine the water, honey and yeast in a jug and set aside for 5–10 minutes. The mixture should start to froth, but don't worry if it doesn't as the bread still bakes well.

In a mixing bowl, combine the flours, salt, spice blend and caraway seeds. Make a well in the centre, then pour in the olive oil and the yeast mixture. Stir until the dough comes together, then transfer to a lightly floured work surface and knead for 10–15 minutes until smooth and elastic. Transfer to a large bowl, cover loosely with plastic wrap and stand in a warm place for 1½ hours or until the bread rises by a little less than half.

Preheat the oven to 220°C (425°F). Line a baking tray with baking paper.

Punch down the dough using your fist, then transfer to a lightly floured work surface and knead for another 3–4 minutes. Shape the dough into a round and place on the prepared tray, tucking the seam underneath. Using a small sharp knife, make several shallow cuts in the top of the dough and lightly brush with water. Sprinkle with the extra caraway seeds. Cover loosely with plastic wrap and stand for another 30 minutes or until slightly risen.

Bake the bread for 10 minutes, then reduce the oven temperature to 180°C (350°F) and bake for another 30 minutes. Remove from the oven and set aside to cool, but not too much, as this bread is best enjoyed warm.

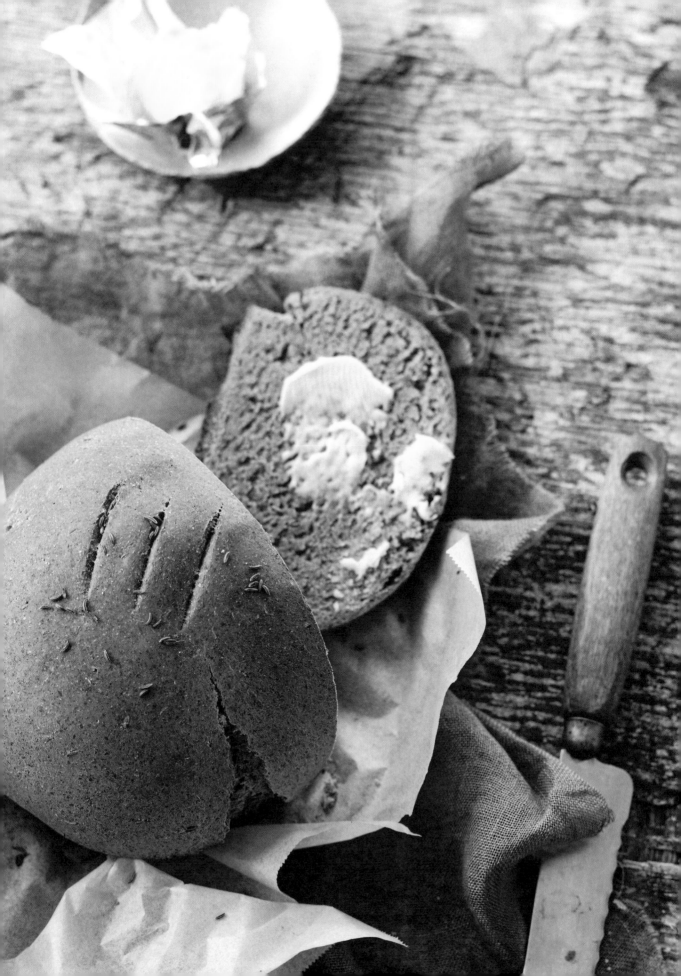

MASH THREE WAYS

+ VEGETARIAN
+ GLUTEN-FREE
+ PALEO

PREP TIME:
10 minutes

COOKING TIME:
25 minutes

BEETROOT & HORSERADISH

Horseradish gives a little kick of flavour.

SERVES 2

1 beetroot (beet), peeled and cut into 1 cm
  (⅜ inch) pieces
2 sebago potatoes, peeled and cut into 2 cm
  (¾ inch) pieces
1 tablespoon finely grated fresh horseradish
¼ teaspoon pink Himalayan salt
2 tablespoons goat's milk yoghurt (or plain
  Greek-style yoghurt)
1 tablespoon chopped toasted almond kernels
1 tablespoon chopped dill

Place the beetroot and potato in a saucepan,
cover with lightly salted cold water and
bring to the boil over high heat. Reduce
the heat to medium and simmer for
20–25 minutes until tender.

Drain well, then mash until smooth. Stir in
the horseradish, salt and yoghurt. Transfer to
a serving dish, scatter with the almonds and
dill and serve immediately.

+ **NOTE** Vegie mash is a delicious way to
  increase your vegetable intake and it's full
  of fibre too.

+ VEGETARIAN
+ VEGAN
+ GLUTEN-FREE
+ DAIRY-FREE
+ PALEO

PREP TIME:
10 minutes

COOKING TIME:
10 minutes

CAULIFLOWER & BROCCOLI

Add healthy fat with creamy avocado.

SERVES 2

90 g (3¼ oz) broccoli (about 1 small head), chopped
120 g (4¼ oz) cauliflower, chopped
1 large kale leaf, finely chopped, stalk removed (about 1 cup)
1 avocado, halved, skin and stone discarded
1 teaspoon lemon juice
¼ teaspoon salt
1 tablespoon chopped mint
2 tablespoons crumbled feta cheese

Put the broccoli and cauliflower into a saucepan of lightly salted boiling water and cook for 7 minutes or until tender. Add the kale and cook for another minute, then drain, reserving 2 tablespoons of the cooking water to thin the mash if necessary.

Transfer the drained vegetables to a blender. Add the avocado, lemon juice and salt and blend until smooth, adding a little of the reserved cooking water if necessary. Scoop into a bowl, scatter with the mint and feta and serve immediately.

+ VEGETARIAN
+ VEGAN
+ GLUTEN-FREE
+ DAIRY-FREE
+ PALEO

PREP TIME:
10 minutes

COOKING TIME:
25 minutes

SPICY CINNAMON SWEET POTATO

Sweet and spicy; great with fish.

SERVES 2

1 large sweet potato (about 450 g/1 lb), peeled and cut into 2 cm (¾ inch) cubes
185 ml (6 fl oz/¾ cup) tinned coconut milk
⅓ teaspoon ground cinnamon
1 pinch salt
1 tablespoon coriander (cilantro) leaves
1 fresh long red chilli, finely chopped (or ½ teaspoon dried chilli flakes)

Put the sweet potato in a saucepan and cover with lightly salted cold water. Bring to the boil over high heat, then reduce the heat to medium and simmer for 20–25 minutes until tender. Drain well.

Put the hot sweet potato in a bowl or jug with the coconut milk, cinnamon and salt and blend with a stick blender until smooth. Scoop into a serving bowl, scatter with the coriander and chilli and serve immediately.

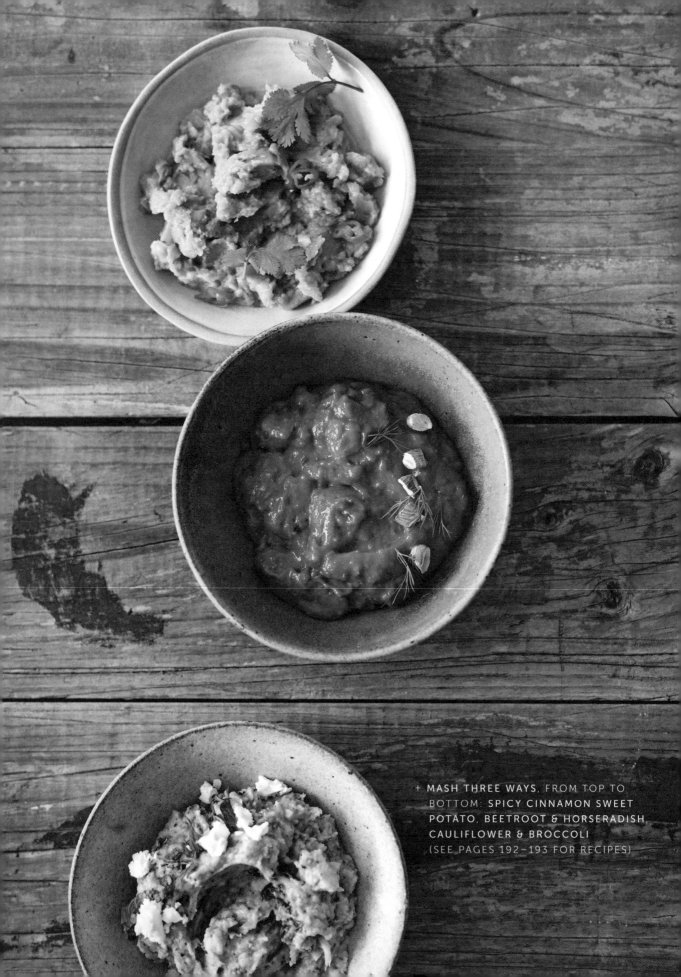

+ MASH THREE WAYS, FROM TOP TO BOTTOM: SPICY CINNAMON SWEET POTATO, BEETROOT & HORSERADISH, CAULIFLOWER & BROCCOLI (SEE PAGES 192–193 FOR RECIPES)

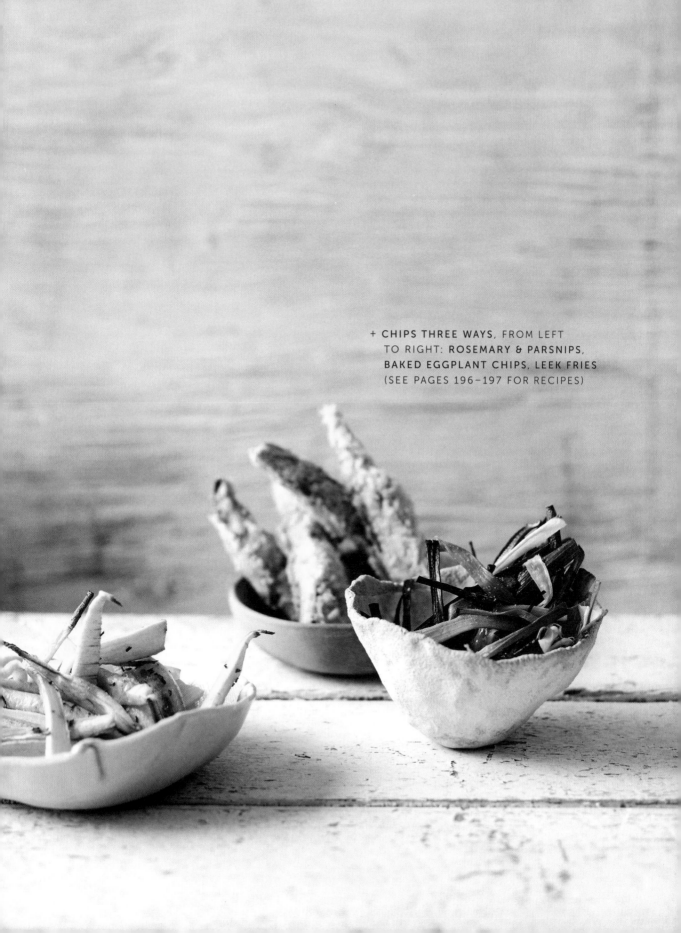

+ CHIPS THREE WAYS, FROM LEFT
TO RIGHT: ROSEMARY & PARSNIPS,
BAKED EGGPLANT CHIPS, LEEK FRIES
(SEE PAGES 196–197 FOR RECIPES)

CHIPS THREE WAYS

+ VEGETARIAN
+ VEGAN
+ GLUTEN-FREE
+ DAIRY-FREE
+ PALEO

PREP TIME:
5 minutes

COOKING TIME:
30 minutes

LEEK FRIES

*Eat these as a snack or add them
to your salads.*

SERVES 1–2

1 leek
1 tablespoon olive oil
½ teaspoon each sea salt and freshly ground
    black pepper

Preheat the oven to 200°C (400°F). Line
a baking tray with baking paper.

Slice the leek in half lengthways, keeping
the root intact, and wash well. Cut each
half into 5–6 cm (2–2½ inch) lengths, then
into 2 cm (¾ inch) wide strips. Spread on
the prepared tray, drizzle with the olive
oil and season with the salt and pepper.
Roast for 20–30 minutes, turning regularly,
until golden.

+ **NOTE** Leeks are milder in flavour than
    onions and have similar health benefits
    to garlic, with antifungal, antibacterial
    and antiviral properties.

+ VEGETARIAN
+ VEGAN
+ GLUTEN-FREE
+ DAIRY-FREE
+ PALEO

PREP TIME:
10 minutes

COOKING TIME:
25 minutes

ROSEMARY & PARSNIPS

Great earthy and nutty flavours. Serve with black olive tapenade or on their own.

SERVES 2

4 parsnips
1 tablespoon olive oil
½ teaspoon salt
1 tablespoon finely chopped rosemary

Preheat the oven to 200°C (400°F). Line a baking tray with baking paper.

Peel the parsnips, cut lengthways into quarters and trim off the woody core. Cut into chips about 5 cm (2 inches) long, then spread on the prepared tray and toss with the remaining ingredients. Roast for 20–25 minutes until golden and tender. Serve hot.

+ **NOTE** Parsnips are sweet root vegetables that look like pale carrots and can also be eaten raw.

+ VEGETARIAN
+ GLUTEN-FREE

PREP TIME:
20 minutes

COOKING TIME:
40 minutes

BAKED EGGPLANT CHIPS

Delicious served with tomato relish or Turmeric Aïoli (see page 166).

SERVES 2

1 eggplant (aubergine)
3 eggs
1 garlic clove, finely chopped
60 g (2¼ oz/½ cup) gluten-free rice breadcrumbs
50 g (1¾ oz/½ cup) grated pecorino cheese
¼ teaspoon cayenne pepper
2 tablespoons olive oil

Preheat oven to 200°C (400°F). Line a baking tray with baking paper. Trim the top off the eggplant and cut into 2 cm (¾ inch) chips.

Whisk the eggs and garlic in a shallow bowl, then combine the breadcrumbs, pecorino, cayenne and a pinch each of salt and pepper in another shallow bowl.

Dip the eggplant chips in the egg mixture and coat with the breadcrumbs. Repeat the dipping and coating process. Spread the chips out on the prepared tray and drizzle with the olive oil. Bake for 40 minutes, turning every 10 minutes until golden on all sides. Sprinkle with a little extra salt and serve immediately.

SNACKS

+ VEGETARIAN
+ VEGAN
+ GLUTEN-FREE
+ DAIRY-FREE
+ PALEO

ZESTY MACADAMIAS

These macadamias are particularly good for snacking. The combination of lime zest and thyme is delicious.

MAKES 1 CUP (2 SERVES)

155 g (5½ oz/1 cup) raw
* macadamia nuts*
1 teaspoon melted coconut oil
¼ teaspoon pink Himalayan salt
1 teaspoon thyme leaves
1 teaspoon lime zest

Preheat the oven to 200°C (400°F). Line a baking tray with baking paper.

Put all of the ingredients in a bowl and stir until well combined. Spread the macadamias over the prepared tray and bake for 8–10 minutes until golden. Remove from the oven and serve warm or at room temperature.

Zesty macadamias can be stored in an airtight container for up to 2 weeks.

+ **NOTE** Coconut oil is a good choice for baking at higher temperatures as it has a very high smoking point and will not burn.

+ VEGETARIAN
+ GLUTEN-FREE
+ PALEO

PREP TIME:
15 minutes

COOKING TIME:
30 minutes

SUPERFOOD CRACKERS

These cheesy, nutty crackers are delicious as a snack or an accompaniment to dips and spreads. For a dairy-free version, replace the parmesan cheese with an extra tablespoon of yeast flakes.

MAKES ABOUT 30 CRACKERS

45 g (1½ oz/¼ cup) chia seeds
75 g (2¾ oz/½ cup) sunflower
    seeds
½ teaspoon thyme leaves
½ teaspoon dried oregano
70 g (2½ oz/½ cup) almond
    kernels
75 g (2¾ oz/½ cup) brazil nuts
25 g (1 oz/¼ cup) LSA meal
    (linseed, sunflower seed
    and almond meal)
2 teaspoons baking powder
50 g (1¾ oz/½ cup) finely grated
    parmesan cheese
2 tablespoons savoury yeast
    flakes
1 tablespoon black tahini
¼ teaspoon each salt and freshly
    ground black pepper
1 egg
1 tablespoon sesame seeds

Preheat the oven to 160°C (315°F). Line a baking tray with baking paper.

Put the chia seeds, sunflower seeds, herbs, nuts, LSA meal and baking powder in a food processor and blitz until the mixture resembles fine breadcrumbs. Transfer the mixture to a bowl. Add 1 tablespoon of water and all of the remaining ingredients, except the sesame seeds, and stir until well combined. Spread the mixture over the lined tray until 5 mm (¼ inch) thick. Moisten your hands and use them to press the dough down.

Run a sharp knife over the mixture to mark squares, so the baked crackers will snap into neat shapes. Sprinkle the sesame seeds over the top, then bake for 30 minutes or until crisp. Remove from the oven and allow to cool on the tray.

These crackers will keep for up to 10 days in an airtight container.

+ **NOTE** Savoury yeast flakes add a cheesy flavour and are high in vitamin B. This is a good vitamin for when you feel run down and stressed.

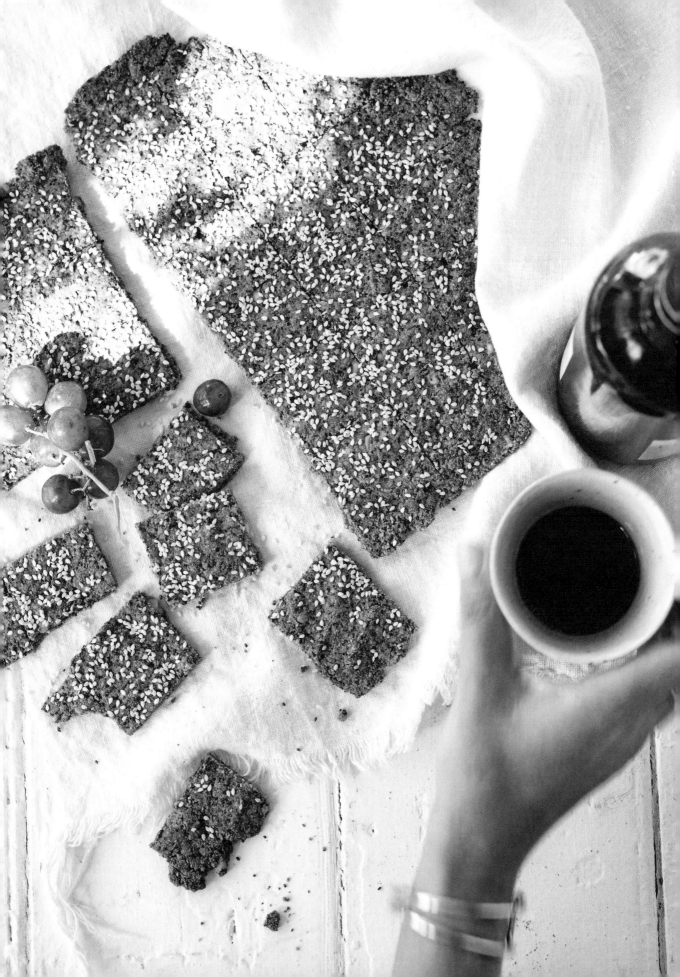

+ VEGETARIAN
+ VEGAN
+ GLUTEN-FREE
+ DAIRY-FREE

SMOKY CHICKPEAS

*My favourite time to eat these is to satisfy the
afternoon munchies. The fibre and protein content
will keep you happy until dinner time.*

MAKES 2 CUPS

*2 x 400 g (14 oz) tins chickpeas,
    drained and rinsed
2 tablespoons macadamia oil
1 teaspoon pink Himalayan salt
1 tablespoon white chia seeds
1½ tablespoons smoked paprika*

Preheat the oven to 150°C (300°F). Line a baking tray
with baking paper.

Put all of the ingredients in a bowl and stir to
combine well. Spread over the prepared tray and
bake for 20–30 minutes until crisp.

Store chickpeas in an airtight container for up to 1 week.

+ **NOTE** Chickpeas are an excellent source of protein
in a vegetarian diet.

LEMON & THYME GRANOLA

Yum! Great for salads and as a topping for fish or a crust for chicken or other meat.

MAKES 6 CUPS

200 g (7 oz/1 cup) white quinoa, rinsed not cooked

75 g (2¾ oz/½ cup) black sesame seeds

75 g (2¾ oz/½ cup) white sesame seeds

40 g (1½ oz/¼ cup) pepitas (pumpkin seeds)

1 teaspoon cayenne pepper

130 g (4½ oz/1 cup) barley flakes

160 g (5¾ oz/1½ cups) instant oats

1 tablespoon dried sage

2 tablespoons thyme leaves

2 tablespoons melted coconut oil

2 tablespoons tahini

Zest of 2 lemons

80 g (2¾ oz/½ cup) linseeds (flaxseeds)

155 g (5½ oz/1 cup) raw macadamia nuts

Preheat the oven to 150°C (300°F). Line a baking tray with baking paper.

Put all of the ingredients in a bowl and combine well. Spread the mixture evenly over the prepared tray and bake, stirring occasionally, for 30 minutes or until golden. Remove from the oven, stand until cool, then store in an airtight container for up to 1 month.

+ **NOTE** Barley flakes are made from the whole grain and have lots of fibre. You can include them in soups and salads as well.

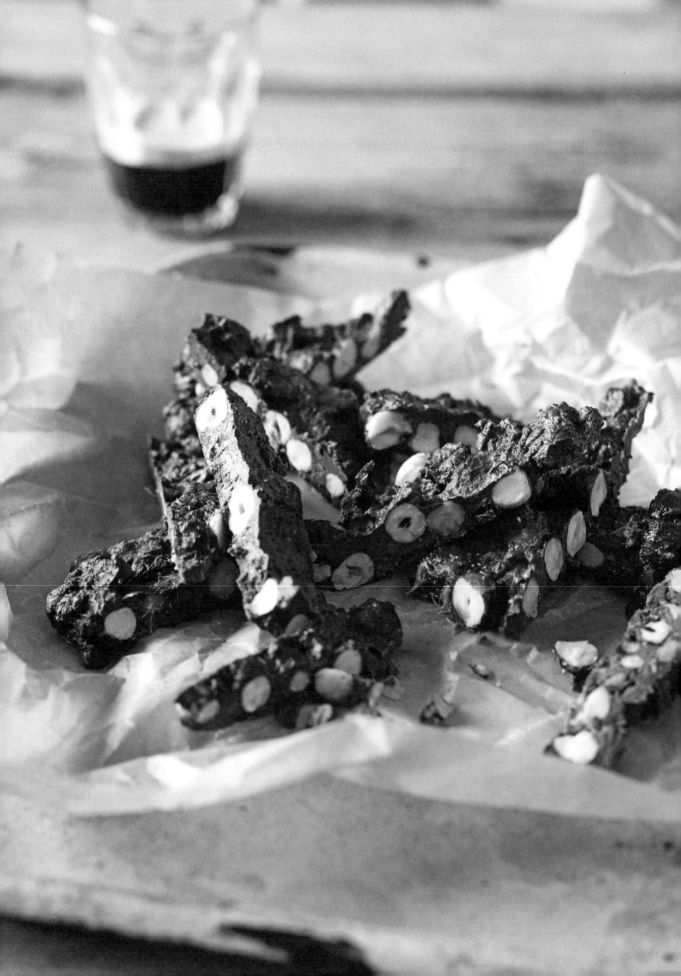

+ VEGETARIAN
+ VEGAN
+ GLUTEN-FREE
+ DAIRY-FREE
+ RAW

PREP TIME:
*15 minutes,
plus 40 minutes
freezing*

COOKING TIME:
15 minutes

HAZELNUT & GINGER CHOCOLATE FUDGE BARK

Who doesn't love hazelnuts and chocolate? It reminds me of my childhood, although I have added a bit of ginger just for that little extra spice. Lovely on its own or served with creamy vanilla ice cream or a fresh cup of organic coffee.

SERVES 4–6

210 g (7½ oz/1½ cups) raw hazelnuts
5 dates, pitted
3 teaspoons white chia seeds
40 g (1½ oz/⅓ cup) cacao powder
25 g (1 oz/¼ cup) LSA meal (linseed, sunflower seed and almond meal)
125 ml (4 fl oz/½ cup) tinned coconut milk
60 ml (2 fl oz/¼ cup) melted coconut oil, plus 1 teaspoon extra
50 g (1¾ oz/¼ cup) peeled and coarsely chopped fresh ginger
3 teaspoons raw honey, or use vegan sweetener

Preheat the oven to 200°C (400°F). Line a baking tray with baking paper and spread the hazelnuts on the tray. Roast for 8–10 minutes until they start to change colour. Remove from the oven and set aside.

Meanwhile, combine the dates, chia seeds, cacao powder, LSA, coconut milk, coconut oil and 1 tablespoon of water in a blender and blend until smooth.

Put the extra teaspoon of coconut oil and the chopped ginger into a small saucepan over medium heat. Stir for 3 minutes or until the ginger begins to turn golden. Add the honey and cook for another 2 minutes or until it begins to crystallise. Remove from the heat, add the toasted hazelnuts and combine well.

Transfer to a mixing bowl, add the date fudge and stir to combine, then spread the mixture over a tray lined with baking paper into a thin square. Place in the freezer for about 30–40 minutes or until set hard. To serve, break up into shards or slice into rough pieces.

HIGH PROTEIN STICKY CHEWY MATCHA BITES

Have these little afternoon snacks with your favourite cup of tea or hot drink; they are sweet and a little salty.

MAKES 12 PIECES

8 dates, pitted and chopped
135 g (4¾ oz/1 cup) ABC nut mix (almonds, brazil nuts and cashews), roughly chopped
20 g (¾ oz/½ cup) coconut chips
40 g (1½ oz/¼ cup) sunflower seeds
60 g (2¼ oz/½ cup) goji berries
¼ teaspoon pink Himalayan salt
2 teaspoons protein powder
2 teaspoons white chia seeds
140 g (5 oz/½ cup) almond butter
2 tablespoons matcha (powdered green tea)
12 goji berries, extra, for decoration

Blend all of the ingredients, except the almond butter, matcha and extra goji berries, in a high-speed blender. Transfer to a mixing bowl, add the almond butter and stir until well combined.

Transfer the mixture to a tray lined with baking paper and use your hands to form the mixture into a square shape about 2 cm (¾ inch) thick. Cut into 12 squares and refrigerate for 20 minutes or until firm.

To serve, dust with matcha and place a goji berry on each bite.

+ **NOTE** Matcha is powdered green tea and is high in Oxygen Radical Absorbance Capacity (ORAC). It's a great pick-me-up with a slow release of caffeine and it also contains theanine, which has a focusing, calming effect on the body. It's perfect for a snack on a busy day.

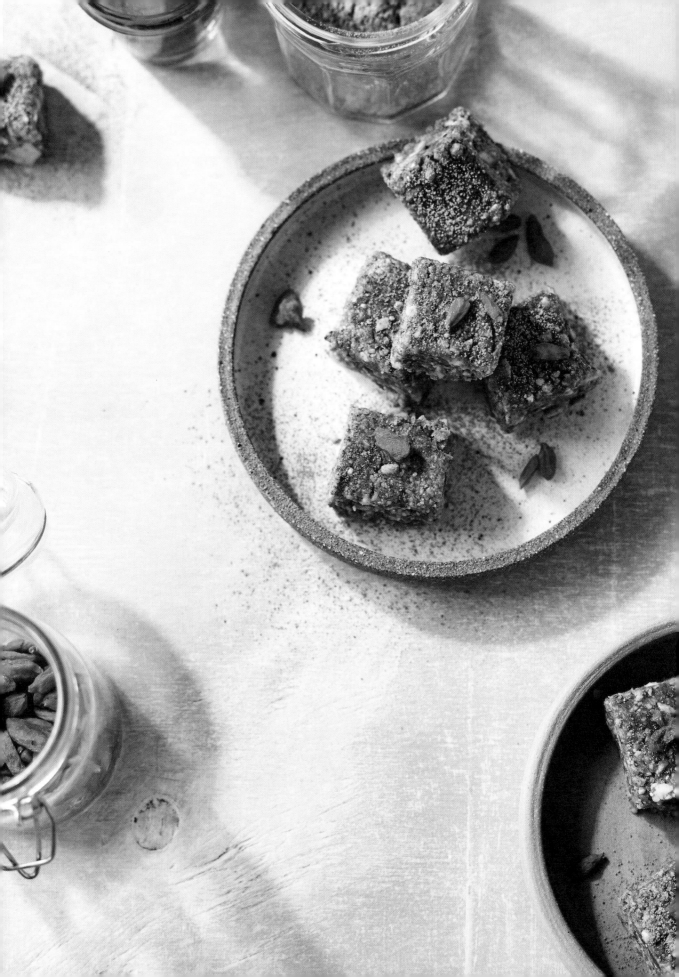

SWEETS

+ VEGETARIAN
+ VEGAN
+ GLUTEN-FREE
+ DAIRY-FREE
+ PALEO
+ RAW

PREP TIME:
20 minutes

COOKING TIME:
Nil

QUINOA CHIA JAM DROPS

A nutritious, low glycaemic index (GI) snack that has been a popular recipe since I first published it. I hope you enjoy it again.

MAKES 12

10 dates, pitted
60 ml (2 fl oz/¼ cup) warm water
150 g (5½ oz/1½ cups) quinoa
 flakes
1 tablespoon shredded coconut
Zest of ½ orange
½ teaspoon ground cinnamon
¼ teaspoon pink Himalayan salt
260 g (9¼ oz/1 cup) almond butter
60 ml (2 fl oz/¼ cup) orange juice
1½ tablespoons Raw Raspberry
 Chia Jam (see page 68)

Soak the dates in the warm water for 10–15 minutes until soft. Transfer the dates and the soaking water to a blender and process until smooth.

Combine the quinoa flakes, coconut, orange zest, cinnamon and salt in a large bowl. Add the almond butter, orange juice and date purée and stir until a smooth, well-combined dough forms. Shape heaped teaspoons of mixture into balls, then place on a tray lined with baking paper. Gently press a thumb into the centre of each ball, then spoon ½ teaspoon of jam into each thumb depression.

These jam drops will keep for up to 10 days in an airtight container in the fridge.

+ **NOTE** Quinoa is a gluten-free seed that is high in protein. Using it in flake form is convenient as it doesn't require cooking. Add quinoa flakes to gluten-free soaked muesli.

+ VEGETARIAN
+ VEGAN
+ GLUTEN-FREE
+ DAIRY-FREE
+ RAW

PREP TIME:
15 minutes, plus
45 minutes chilling

COOKING TIME:
Nil

RAW ROCKY ROAD

*Instead of marshmallows, opt for crunchy
macadamias combined with sour cherries
for a perfectly balanced flavour.*

MAKES ABOUT 15 PIECES

*625 ml (21½ fl oz/2½ cups) melted
    coconut oil*
55 g (2 oz/½ cup) cacao powder
1 pinch salt
*310 ml (10¾ fl oz/1¼ cups) pure
    maple syrup*
200 g (7 oz/2 cups) almond meal
*110 g (3¾ oz/2 cups) coconut
    flakes*
*120 g (4¼ oz/1 cup) coarsely
    chopped macadamia nuts*
120 g (4¼ oz/1 cup) goji berries
*85 g (3 oz/½ cup) dried sour
    cherries, chopped*

Lightly grease a 34 x 24 cm (13½ x 9½ inch) baking tin and line it with baking paper, leaving the sides overhanging.

Put the coconut oil, cacao powder, salt, maple syrup and almond meal in a bowl and stir until well combined. Add the remaining ingredients and stir until well combined. Spoon into the prepared tin and refrigerate for 45 minutes or until set. Cut into slices to serve.

This rocky road will keep for about 3 weeks in an airtight container in the fridge.

+ **NOTE** Sour cherries, packed with antivirals and anti-inflammatories, are zingy little taste bombs.

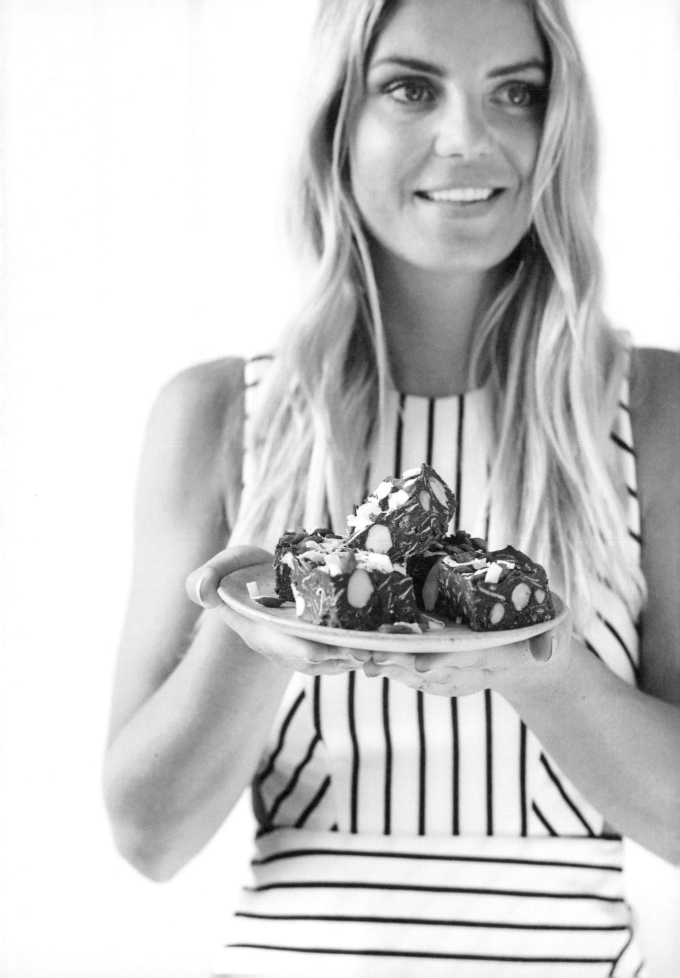

+ GLUTEN-FREE
+ DAIRY-FREE

PREP TIME:
*10 minutes, plus
2 hours chilling*

COOKING TIME:
5 minutes

VANILLA & MAPLE GUT-HEALING MARSHMALLOWS

*Tasty as a snack or with a cup of hot chocolate
and very healing: two birds, one stone!*

MAKES 32

*3 tablespoons grass-fed bovine
    gelatine powder
500 ml (17 fl oz/2 cups) tinned
    coconut milk
1 teaspoon vanilla bean paste
2 tablespoons pure maple syrup*

Put the gelatine in a small bowl with 80 ml
(2½ fl oz/⅓ cup) of cold water and stir until
well combined.

Heat the coconut milk in a saucepan over low to
medium heat until just below boiling point. Remove
from the heat and stir in the vanilla bean paste and
maple syrup. Add the gelatine and stir vigorously until
all is well combined. Pour the mixture into two silicone
icetrays, then refrigerate for 2 hours or until firm.
If you don't have silicone icetrays, very lightly grease
a standard icetray with coconut or almond oil before
pouring in the marshmallow mixture. This will make
it easier to remove the marshmallows when set.

These marshmallows will keep for 10 days in an airtight
container in the fridge.

+ **NOTE** Grass-fed bovine gelatine powder is premium-
    quality gelatine from healthy animals. Gelatine's high
    amino-acid content supports a healthy mood, strong
    bones, smooth skin and proper muscle synthesis. It is
    also great for gut support.

+ VEGETARIAN
+ VEGAN
+ GLUTEN-FREE
+ DAIRY-FREE
+ RAW

PREP TIME:
20 minutes, plus
2 hours soaking
and 1 hour freezing

COOKING TIME:
Nil

RAW CHERRY CHOC SLICE

Just like a chocolate bar, but better for you.

MAKES 15 PIECES

BASE
160 g (5¾ oz/1 cup) pitted dates
440 g (15½ oz/2¾ cups) almond
    kernels
½ teaspoon natural vanilla extract
55 g (2 oz/½ cup) cacao powder

CHERRY LAYER
120 g (4¼ oz/¾ cup) raw cashews
360 g (12¾ oz/3 cups) frozen sour
    cherries
60 g (2¼ oz/½ cup) frozen
    raspberries
170 ml (5½ fl oz/⅔ cup) pure
    maple syrup
125 ml (4 fl oz/½ cup) melted
    coconut oil
1 pinch salt
225 g (8 oz/2½ cups) desiccated
    coconut

CHOCOLATE LAYER
80 g (2¾ oz/¾ cup) cacao powder
1½ teaspoons carob powder
310 ml (10¾ fl oz/1¼ cups) melted
    coconut oil
2 tablespoons tinned coconut milk

Soak the raw cashews for the cherry layer in cold water for 2 hours. Drain well before using.

To make the base, put all of the ingredients in a blender, add 2 tablespoons of water and process until coarsely chopped. Turn the mixture into a lightly greased 34 x 24 cm (13½ x 9½ inch) baking tin and press down with the palm of your hand until the mixture covers the base of the tin in an even layer.

To make the cherry layer, process all of the ingredients in a blender until coarsely chopped. Pour over the base, then freeze for 30 minutes or until set.

To make the chocolate layer, process all of the ingredients in a blender until smooth. Pour over the cherry layer, then return to the freezer for another 30 minutes or until set, then cut into slices.

This slice will keep for up to 3 weeks in an airtight container in the fridge.

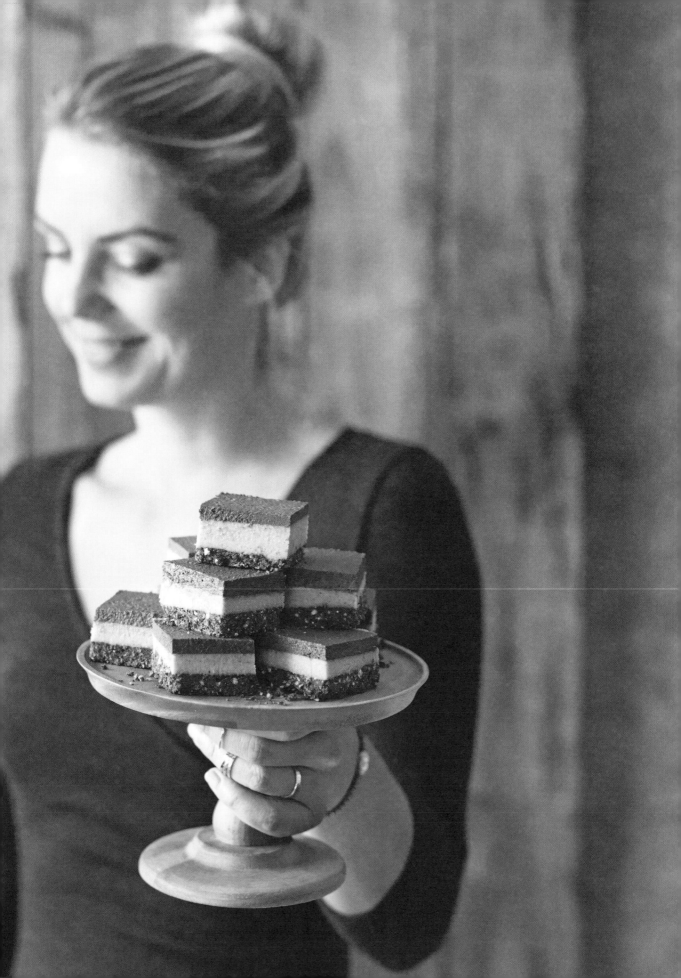

PREP TIME:
*30 minutes, plus
2 hours soaking and
45 minutes freezing*

COOKING TIME:
Nil

RAW PEPPERMINT SLICE

This decadent slice is one of our best sellers.

MAKES 15 PIECES

195 g (6¾ oz/1 cup) buckwheat
    kernels
75 g (2¾ oz/⅔ cup) cacao powder
100 g (3½ oz/1 cup) pecans
160 g (3½ oz/1 cup) pitted dates
2 tablespoons melted coconut oil
1 pinch salt

PEPPERMINT CREAM
275 g (9¾ oz/1¾ cups) raw cashews
185 ml (6 fl oz/¾ cup) pure maple
    syrup
250 ml (9 fl oz/1 cup) melted
    coconut oil
170 ml (5½ fl oz/⅔ cup) melted
    coconut butter
1 teaspoon natural vanilla extract
1 pinch spirulina powder
1 teaspoon liquid chlorophyll
1 pinch salt
1 teaspoon peppermint oil

CHOCOLATE GANACHE
195 g (6¾ oz/1¼ cups) raw cashews
250 ml (9 fl oz/1 cup) melted
    coconut oil
125 ml (4 fl oz/½ cup) maple syrup
80 g (2¾ oz/¾ cup) cacao powder
½ teaspoon natural vanilla extract

Soak the raw cashews for the peppermint cream and ganache in cold water for 2 hours. Drain before using.

To make the base, process all of the ingredients in a blender until coarsely chopped. Turn the mixture into a lightly greased 34 x 24 cm (13½ x 9½ inch) baking tin and press down with the palm of your hand until the mixture covers the base of the tin in an even layer.

To make the peppermint cream layer, process all of the ingredients in a blender until smooth, then pour on top of the base and spread with a spatula until smooth. Freeze for 15 minutes or until set.

To make the ganache, process all of the ingredients in a blender until smooth. Pour the ganache over the peppermint layer and spread with a spatula until smooth. Return to the freezer for another 30 minutes or until set.

The slice will keep for up to 3 weeks, refrigerated or frozen in an airtight container.

+ **NOTE** Buckwheat has a really nutty and earthy flavour. There's just something wholesome about this grain, and it's great for people who are sensitive to wheat (funny that, given the name!) and other gluten grains. It is mostly used in rice-like dishes.

+ VEGETARIAN
+ GLUTEN-FREE
+ PALEO

PREP TIME:
20 minutes

COOKING TIME:
1½ hours

BEST-EVER BANANA BREAD

This banana bread is super-yummy, moist and light. Grain-free, it just ticks all the boxes for me. I've called it the best ever because, when I first published the recipe, the comments on social media went wild!

SERVES 6 (MAKES 1 LOAF)

4 bananas, sliced
125 ml (4 fl oz/½ cup) pure maple syrup
7 eggs
1 tablespoon vanilla bean paste
330 g (11¾ oz/1¼ cups) almond butter
100 g (3½ oz/¾ cup) coconut flour
1 tablespoon baking powder
1 tablespoon bicarbonate of soda (baking soda)
1 tablespoon ground cinnamon
1 teaspoon pink Himalayan salt

TOPPING
2 tablespoons unsalted butter, softened
2 tablespoons coconut sugar
1 tablespoon ground cinnamon
25 g (1 oz/¼ cup) almond meal
85 g (3 oz/⅔ cup) chopped pecans

Preheat the oven to 160°C (315°F). Grease a 30 x 12 x 10 cm (12 x 4½ x 4 inch) loaf (bar) tin and line it with baking paper, leaving the sides overhanging.

Put the banana, maple syrup, eggs, vanilla bean paste and almond butter in a large bowl and stir to combine well. Combine the remaining dry ingredients in a separate bowl, then add to the banana mixture and stir until well combined. Pour into the prepared tin.

Put all of the topping ingredients in a bowl and stir until well combined. Sprinkle on top of the batter, then cover the tin with foil or a metal tray and bake for 1 hour. Remove the foil and bake for another 20–30 minutes until a skewer inserted into the centre comes out clean. Remove from the oven and stand until cool, then slice and serve.

+ **NOTE** Coconut sugar is mineral rich and has a low glycaemic index (GI). As an alternative to granulated sugar, it gives a rich toffee flavour to desserts.

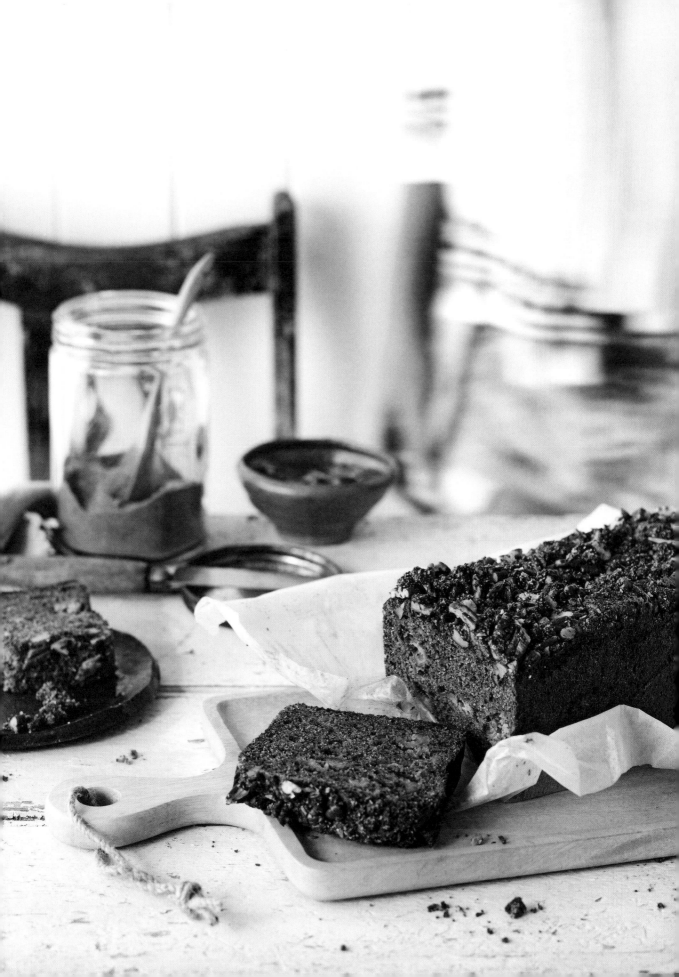

MATCHA LIME MACADAMIA CHEESECAKE

This is a great festive cake that I have made for New Year's Eve parties, where it is a crowd pleaser.

SERVES 6–8

20 g (¾ oz/¼ cup) shredded coconut
Chopped salted macadamia nuts and lime segments, to serve

BASE
230 g (8¼ oz/1½ cups) raw macadamia nuts
2 tablespoons rice malt syrup
1 tablespoon macadamia nut butter
65 g (2½ oz/1 cup) shredded coconut
1 tablespoon vanilla bean paste
¼ teaspoon pink Himalayan salt
60 ml (2 fl oz/¼ cup) melted coconut oil
2 tablespoons lime juice

FILLING
3 ripe avocados, halved, skin and stones discarded
125 ml (4 fl oz/½ cup) tinned coconut milk
125 ml (4 fl oz/½ cup) lime juice
2 teaspoons finely grated lime zest
2 tablespoons rice malt syrup
45 g (1½ oz/¼ cup) chia seeds
3 teaspoons matcha (powdered green tea)

ICING
155 g (5½ oz/1 cup) raw cashews
250 ml (9 fl oz/1 cup) coconut water
60 ml (2 fl oz/¼ cup) lime juice
Juice of 1 lemon
125 ml (4 fl oz/½ cup) coconut cream
125 ml (4 fl oz/½ cup) rice malt syrup
3 tablespoons grass-fed bovine gelatine powder (or chia seeds for a vegan version)

To make the base, put all of the ingredients in a blender and process until well combined. Turn the mixture into a lightly greased 25 cm (10 inch) round springform cake tin. Refrigerate for 20 minutes.

Meanwhile, to make the filling, process all of the ingredients in a blender until smooth and well combined. Pour over the chilled base and refrigerate overnight.

Soak the raw cashews for the icing in cold water for 2 hours. Drain well before using.

To make the icing, put all of the ingredients in a blender and process until smooth and well combined.

To assemble, remove the cheesecake from the tin and place on a cake stand or plate. Spread the icing over the top and cover the side with the shredded coconut. Decorate the top with chopped salted macadamias and lime segments. Refrigerate for 40 minutes or until the icing has set, then cut into slices to serve.

+ NOTE Lime has an irresistible scent, which makes the mouth water. This is where digestion starts.

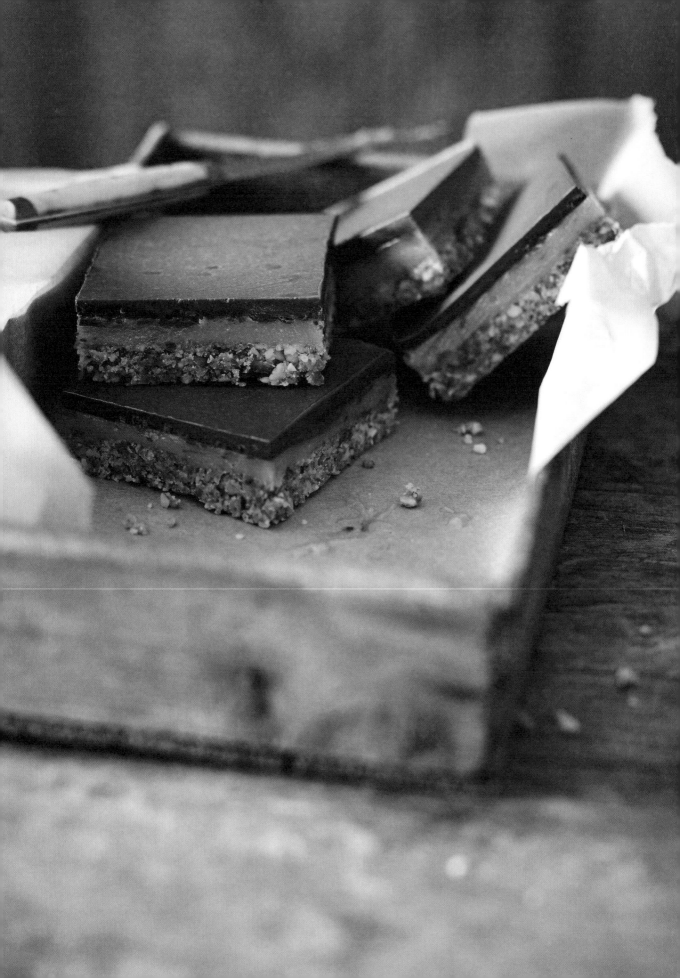

+ VEGETARIAN
+ VEGAN
+ GLUTEN-FREE
+ DAIRY-FREE
+ RAW

PREP TIME:
*25 minutes, plus
45 minutes freezing*

COOKING TIME:
Nil

RAW CARAMEL SLICE

*This is a naughty but nice kind of treat and it's
no wonder that it's on our bestsellers list week
after week! The creaminess from the tahini adds
real caramel flavour.*

MAKES 12 PIECES

BASE
160 g (5¾ oz/1 cup) pitted dates
*440 g (15½ oz/2¾ cups) almond
    kernels*
*½ teaspoon natural vanilla
    extract*

CARAMEL LAYER
205 g (7¼ oz/¾ cup) tahini
*250 ml (9 fl oz/1 cup) pure maple
    syrup*
*125 ml (4 fl oz/½ cup) melted
    coconut oil*
*2 teaspoons natural vanilla
    extract*
1 pinch salt

TOPPING
80 g (2¾ oz/¾ cup) cacao powder
1½ tablespoons carob powder
*250 ml (9 fl oz/1 cup) melted
    coconut oil*
2 tablespoons tinned coconut milk

To make the base, put all of the ingredients into a
blender with 2 tablespoons of water and blend until
coarsely chopped. Turn the mixture into a lightly
greased 34 x 24 cm (13½ x 9½ inch) baking tin and press
down with the palm of your hand until the mixture
covers the base of the tin in an even layer.

To make the caramel layer, combine all the ingredients
in a bowl and stir until smooth. Pour into the tin over
the base and freeze for 15 minutes or until set.

To make the topping, put all of the ingredients in
a bowl and stir until well combined. Pour into the
tin over the caramel layer and return to the freezer
for another 30 minutes or until set. Cut into 12 pieces.

This slice will keep for about 3 weeks in an airtight
container in the fridge.

+ **NOTE** Dates are a sweet substitute for sugar and, as
    they are easily digested, they make a great afternoon
    snack. Try them with almond butter or peanut butter!

PREP TIME:
40 minutes, plus
overnight soaking

COOKING TIME:
40 minutes

MAKOVÁ TORTA WITH SOUR CHERRY SORBET & RAW CACAO GANACHE

I come from a land where poppy seeds are a staple in baking and desserts, so for nostalgia I love to add these crunchy little pips to desserts. I have used cherries in this recipe, as I usually make this cake at Christmas time. Cherries are in season for such a small window of time, but you can substitute blueberries and raspberries for the cherries at other times of the year.

SERVES 6–8

235 g (8½ oz/1½ cups) poppy seeds
250 ml (9 fl oz/1 cup) almond milk
Coconut oil, for greasing
150 g (5½ oz) unsalted butter, softened
1 teaspoon vanilla bean paste
85 g (3 oz) coconut sugar
5 eggs, separated
150 g (5½ oz/1½ cups) almond meal
1 teaspoon baking powder
¼ teaspoon pink Himalayan salt
Fresh cherries or seasonal berries, and edible flowers (optional), to serve

ORANGE AND LEMON FILLING
95 g (3¼ oz/⅓ cup) Greek-style yoghurt
Juice of ½ lemon

Juice and zest of 1 orange
40 g (1½ oz/¼ cup) poppy seeds
2 teaspoons coconut sugar
3 teaspoons grass-fed bovine gelatine powder

SOUR CHERRY SORBET
2 cups frozen sour cherries
50 g (1¾ oz/¼ cup) coconut sugar
125 ml (4 fl oz/½ cup) coconut cream

RAW CACAO GANACHE
30 g (1 oz/¼ cup) cacao powder
125 ml (4 fl oz/½ cup) tinned coconut milk
5 teaspoons chia seeds
150 g (5½ oz/1 cup) fresh pitted cherries or other berries

Continued overleaf

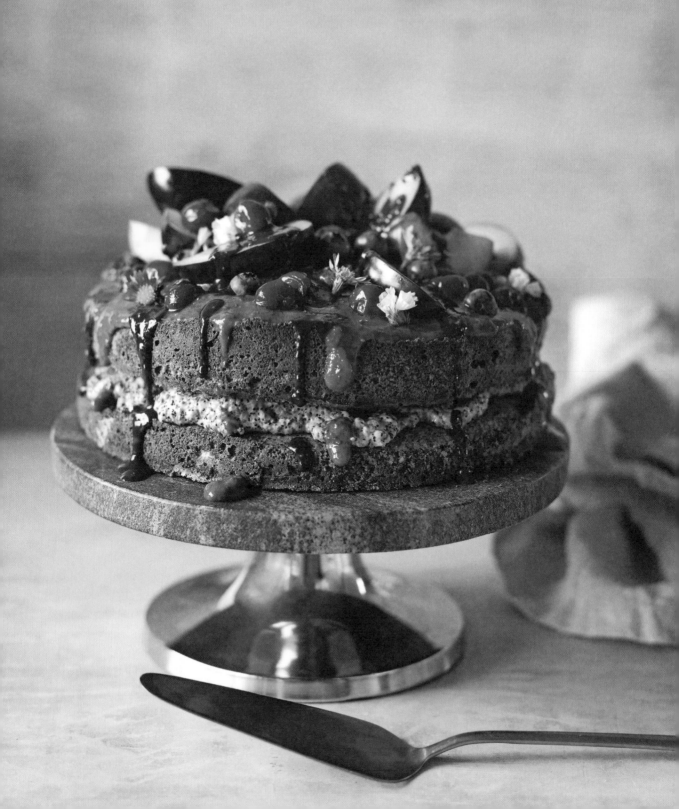

Soak the poppy seeds in the almond milk overnight. Drain the poppy seeds and discard the liquid.

Preheat the oven to 180°C (350°F). Lightly grease two 18 cm (7 inch) round cake tins with coconut oil and line the bases with baking paper.

Using a stand mixer fitted with the whisk attachment, beat the butter, vanilla bean paste and coconut sugar until pale and fluffy. Beat in the egg yolks one at a time. Stir in the almond meal, baking powder, salt and the drained poppy seeds.

Put the egg whites in a spotlessly clean bowl and whisk until stiff peaks form. Fold one-third of the egg whites into the batter to loosen, then fold in the remaining egg whites until just combined. Divide the batter between the prepared tins and bake for 40 minutes or until a skewer inserted into the centre comes out clean. Allow to cool in the tins for 5 minutes, then turn out onto a wire rack to cool completely.

Meanwhile, to make the filling, whisk all of the ingredients together until well combined, then set aside for 15 minutes.

To make the sorbet, combine all of the ingredients in a high-speed blender and process to combine.

To make the ganache, put all of the ingredients in a bowl and whisk until well combined. Refrigerate for 10 minutes to firm up slightly.

To assemble the cake, place one of the cakes on a cake stand. Spread the orange and lemon filling over the top, then place the second cake on top and cover with the sour cherry sorbet. Decorate with fresh cherries, seasonal fruit and edible flowers (if using), then drizzle the ganache over the top.

The torta is best eaten on the day of making, but will keep for 2–3 days in an airtight container in the fridge.

+ **NOTE** Poppy seeds are rich in essential fatty acids and also in calcium, potassium, phosphorus and magnesium. Poppy seeds also contain high levels of vitamin B, folic acid, thiamin and riboflavin. They are a great addition to baked and raw desserts, salads, smoothies and as a crust on fish or chicken.

PREP TIME:
20 minutes

COOKING TIME:
5 minutes

TIRAMISU CUPS

A nutritious spin on a classic dessert.

SERVES 4

135 g (4¾ oz/1 cup) raw hazelnuts
125 g (4½ oz/1 cup) fresh
   raspberries

BISCUIT CRUMB
100 g (3½ oz/1 cup) almond meal
8 dates, pitted
1 teaspoon vanilla bean paste
1 tablespoon finely ground
   coffee beans

QUARK MIX
200 g (7 oz/1 cup) quark (or use
   Greek-style yoghurt)
2 teaspoons vanilla bean paste
2 teaspoons pure maple syrup

CACAO GANACHE
1 ripe avocado, halved
   lengthways, skin and
   stone discarded
2 teaspoons chia seeds
1 tablespoon cacao powder
2 tablespoons coconut cream
1 tablespoon pure maple syrup
Double shot of freshly brewed
   espresso coffee

Put the hazelnuts in a dry frying pan and shake over medium heat for 2–3 minutes until lightly toasted. Set aside to cool, then coarsely chop.

Meanwhile, to make the biscuit crumb, combine all of the ingredients in a high-speed blender and process until finely ground.

To make the quark mix, combine all of the ingredients in a bowl and stir until smooth.

To make the cacao ganache, combine all of the ingredients in a high-speed blender and process until smooth.

To assemble, place 1 tablespoon of the biscuit crumb in the base of each serving cup or glass. Top with 2 tablespoons of the quark mixture, another tablespoon of the biscuit crumbs, another tablespoon of quark mix, then the ganache. At this point you can refrigerate the tiramisu until ready to serve. To serve, top the tiramisu with the hazelnuts and raspberries.

+ VEGETARIAN
+ GLUTEN-FREE
+ PALEO

THUMBPRINT TEFF CACAO COOKIES WITH VANILLA BLUEBERRY JAM

Uncooked teff grains give these cookies crunch.

MAKES 26

120 g (4¼ oz/½ cup) uncooked teff
130 g (4½ oz/1 cup) coconut flour
½ teaspoon pink Himalayan salt
125 ml (4 fl oz/½ cup) pure maple
    syrup
125 ml (4 fl oz/½ cup) melted
    coconut butter
1 teaspoon vanilla bean paste
260 g (9¼ oz/1 cup) almond butter
30 g (1 oz/¼ cup) cacao powder
2 tablespoons cacao nibs
80 g (2¾ oz/½ cup) chopped
    almond kernels
4 eggs, lightly beaten
125 ml (4 fl oz/½ cup) hot water
26 whole almond kernels

VANILLA BLUEBERRY JAM
45 g (1½ oz/¼ cup) white chia
    seeds
½ teaspoon coconut nectar
    (see note)
½ teaspoon vanilla bean paste
155 g (5½ oz/1 cup) fresh or
    defrosted frozen blueberries

Preheat the oven to 180°C (350°F) and line two baking trays with baking paper.

To make the cookies, put all of the ingredients, except the whole almonds, in a large bowl and stir to combine. Shape the mixture into walnut-sized balls and place on the prepared trays, leaving a 3–4 cm (1¼–1¾ inch) space between each one. Gently press your thumb into the centre of each ball. Bake for 25 minutes or until light golden. Allow to cool on the trays.

Meanwhile, to make the jam, put the chia seeds, coconut nectar and 125 ml (4 fl oz/½ cup) of water in a bowl and stand for 15 minutes. Transfer the mixture to a blender, add the vanilla bean paste and blueberries and blitz until smooth. The leftover jam will keep for up to 1 month in an airtight container in the fridge.

Put the whole almonds in a dry frying pan and shake over high heat for 5 minutes or until they start to change colour. Remove from the pan and allow to cool.

Spoon 1 teaspoon of jam into the thumbprint in each cookie, then top with a toasted almond. These cookies will keep for up to 1 week in an airtight container.

+ **NOTE** Coconut nectar has a toffee flavour.

+ VEGETARIAN
+ VEGAN
+ GLUTEN-FREE
+ DAIRY-FREE

PREP TIME:
30 minutes

COOKING TIME:
25 minutes

EGGPLANT BEETROOT BROWNIE WITH SALTED MISO CARAMEL SAUCE

Eggplant gives a creamy texture to this brownie.

SERVES 6–8

1 large eggplant (aubergine)
2 teaspoons coconut oil
250 ml (9 fl oz/1 cup) beetroot juice
100 g (3½ oz) dates, pitted
100 g (3½ oz/½ cup) coconut sugar
50 g (1¾ oz/½ cup) oat flour
160 g (5¾ oz/1 cup) brown rice
   flour
½ teaspoon baking powder
½ teaspoon bicarbonate of soda
   (baking soda)
55 g (2 oz/½ cup) cacao powder
60 g (2¼ oz/½ cup) pecans, chopped
75 g (2¾ oz) dark chocolate (85%
   cocoa solids), coarsely chopped
Fresh blueberries and Greek-style
   yoghurt, to serve

SALTED MISO CARAMEL SAUCE
205 g (7¼ oz/¾ cup) tahini
250 ml (9 fl oz/1 cup) pure maple
   syrup
125 ml (4 fl oz/½ cup) melted
   coconut oil
2 teaspoons natural vanilla
   extract
2 teaspoons white (shiro) miso

Preheat the oven to 160°C (315°F). Lightly grease a 33 cm (13 inch) round cake tin and line the base with baking paper.

Peel the eggplant and cut it into 1 cm (⅜ inch) cubes. Put the coconut oil in a frying pan over medium heat. Add the eggplant and cook for 5 minutes, adding 2 tablespoons of water every minute until the eggplant is soft and the water has evaporated. Transfer the eggplant mixture to a blender, add the beetroot juice and dates and process until smooth.

Combine all of the dry ingredients including the nuts and chocolate in a large bowl and stir to mix well. Add the eggplant mixture and gently stir until smooth. Pour into the prepared tin and bake for 20 minutes or until a skewer inserted into the centre comes out clean. Remove from the oven and allow to cool in the tin.

To make the salted miso caramel sauce, combine all of the ingredients in a bowl with a pinch of salt and stir until smooth. Pour the sauce over the cooled brownie, then scatter with blueberries. Cut into wedges and serve with Greek-style yoghurt.

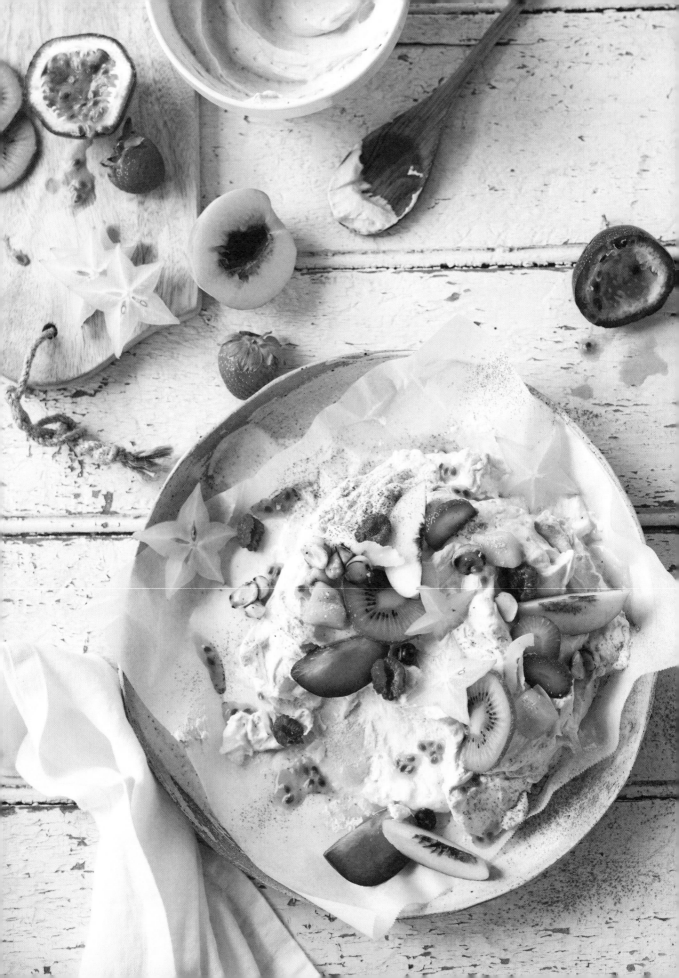

+ VEGETARIAN
+ GLUTEN-FREE
+ PALEO

PREP TIME:
*25 minutes, plus
30 minutes cooling*

COOKING TIME:
20 minutes

GREEN & GOLD PAVLOVA WITH FINGER LIME & MATCHA CREAM

I was inspired to create this green and gold pavlova using Australian finger lime, turmeric and matcha. Go green and gold! Use leftover egg yolks for Chorizo White Bean Frittata (see page 125).

SERVES 4

155 g (5½ oz/1 cup) raw
　　macadamia nuts
1 tablespoon raw honey
300 ml (10½ fl oz) pouring cream
½ teaspoon matcha (powdered
　　green tea)
½ teaspoon finger lime powder
　　(or the zest of 1 lime)
125 g (4½ oz) strawberries, hulled
　　and halved
3 passionfruit
Seasonal fruit, such as peaches,
　　plums, kiwi fruit and star fruit
50 g (1¾ oz/½ cup) flaked
　　almonds, toasted
10 g (⅜ oz/¼ cup) coconut chips,
　　toasted

PAVLOVA
5 egg whites
100 g (3½ oz) honey
1 teaspoon lemon juice
¼ teaspoon ground turmeric
1 tablespoon tapioca starch
　　or flour

Preheat the oven to 140°C (275°F). Line a baking tray with baking paper.

To make the pavlova, use a stand mixer fitted with the whisk attachment to beat the egg whites until stiff peaks form. With the motor running, gradually add the honey, whisking after each addition until soft peaks form. Combine the lemon juice and turmeric in a small bowl, then use a spatula to gently fold into the meringue until just combined. Gently fold in the tapioca starch. Spoon the mixture onto the lined tray to create a 25 cm (10 inch) round, smoothing the sides with a spatula. Bake for 20 minutes or until set. Remove from the oven and stand on the tray until completely cool.

Meanwhile, toast the macadamias in a dry frying pan over high heat for 2 minutes or until golden. Add the honey and cook for another minute until coated. Remove from the heat and allow to cool.

To serve, combine the cream, matcha and finger lime powder in a bowl and whisk until firm peaks form. Place the pavlova on a serving plate, spread the cream over, top with fruit and scatter the almonds, coconut flakes and honey macadamias over the top.

GIANT LAMINGTON WITH RASPBERRY KAKADU JAM

Considered a gift of the Dreamtime, the Kakadu plum is Australia's star superfood. They have exceptional nutritional and antiseptic properties.

SERVES 6–8

6 eggs
115 g (4 oz/⅓ cup) honey
80 ml (2½ fl oz/⅓ cup) melted coconut oil
1 teaspoon vanilla bean paste
65 g (2½ oz/½ cup) coconut flour
½ teaspoon baking powder
100 g (3½ oz/1 cup) almond meal
35 g (1¼ oz/½ cup) shredded coconut

KAKADU JAM
170 g (6 oz) raspberries, fresh or frozen and defrosted
50 g (1¾ oz/¼ cup) coconut sugar
1 tablespoon Kakadu plum (salty plum) powder, or use the zest of 1 orange
45 g (1½ oz/¼ cup) chia seeds
2 tablespoons coconut water

CACAO FROSTING
40 g (1½ oz/¼ cup) coconut oil
55 g (2 oz/½ cup) cacao powder
60 ml (2 fl oz/¼ cup) coconut cream

Preheat the oven to 160°C. Lightly grease a 30 x 12 x 10 cm (12 x 4½ x 4 inch) loaf (bar) tin and line it with baking paper, leaving the sides overhanging.

Use an electric mixer fitted with the whisk attachment to whisk the eggs and honey for 5 minutes or until well combined. Add the coconut oil and vanilla bean paste and whisk for another 2–3 minutes until well combined.

Combine the coconut flour, baking powder and almond meal in a separate bowl. Gently fold into the egg mixture until just combined, then spoon into the prepared tin and bake for 40 minutes or until a skewer comes out clean. Remove from the oven and allow to cool in the tin.

Meanwhile, to make the jam, combine the ingredients in a blender and blend until smooth. Transfer to a small bowl, cover and refrigerate for 15 minutes or until set.

To make cacao frosting, put the coconut oil in a frying pan with 60 ml (2 fl oz/¼ cup) of water and cook over low heat until the oil melts. Add the cacao powder and coconut cream and stir for 2 minutes or until combined. Remove from the heat and set aside to cool.

Transfer the cake to a serving plate. Spread with jam and drizzle with the frosting. Scatter with shredded coconut.

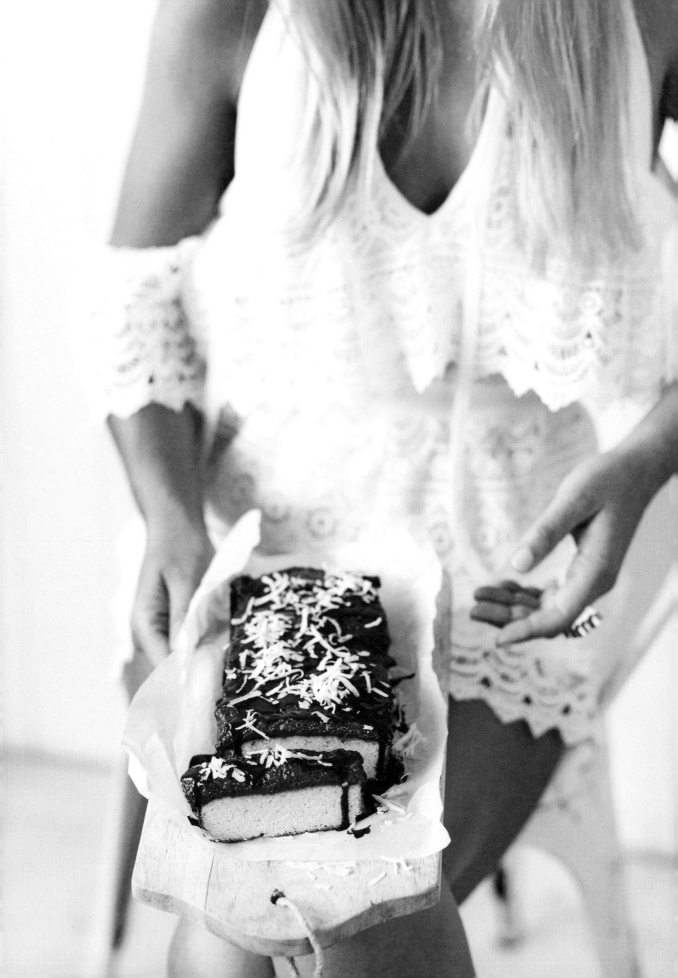

+ VEGETARIAN
+ VEGAN
+ GLUTEN-FREE
+ DAIRY-FREE
+ PALEO
+ RAW

PREP TIME:
10 minutes
COOKING TIME:
Nil

MATCHA ICE CREAM

This recipe is quick and easy. Using frozen banana creates an instant ice cream mousse.

SERVES 2

1 banana, frozen
2 tablespoons almond butter
¼ teaspoon pink Himalayan salt
130 g (4½ oz/½ cup) natural
    yoghurt
2 teaspoons natural vanilla
    extract
1½ tablespoons chia seeds
2 teaspoons matcha (powdered
    green tea)
1 tablespoon maple syrup
Raspberries or other fresh fruit,
    to serve

Combine all of the ingredients in a high-speed blender and process until smooth. Serve immediately in glass jars, topped with fresh fruit.

+ **NOTE** Banana supplies fibre and potassium and is good for the digestion. This fruit literally makes you happy: high levels of tryptophan convert into seratonin, the brain's mood regulator.

+ VEGETARIAN
+ DAIRY-FREE

PREP TIME:
15 minutes

COOKING TIME:
20 minutes

WATTLESEED MACADAMIA CHEWY BARK

This crunchy bark is amazing on its own or served with vanilla ice cream. Wattleseed is a perfect ingredient to pair with an iconic Australian biscuit recipe, given that it can survive tough weather conditions and historically was a valuable source of protein and carbohydrate in times of drought.

SERVES 6–8

170 ml (5½ fl oz/⅔ cup) macadamia oil
2 tablespoons honey
½ teaspoon bicarbonate of soda (baking soda)
1 tablespoon boiling water

DRY MIX
95 g (3¼ oz/1 cup) rolled oats
55 g (2 oz/¾ cup) shredded coconut
60 g (2¼ oz/½ cup) tapioca flour
65 g (2½ oz/½ cup) coconut flour
100 g (3½ oz/½ cup) coconut sugar
2 tablespoons rosemary leaves, chopped
1 tablespoon wattleseed powder
120 g (4¼ oz/1 cup) chopped roasted macadamia nuts

Preheat the oven to 160°C (315°F). Line a large, lightly greased baking tray with baking paper.

Put all of the dry mix ingredients into a bowl and combine well.

Put the macadamia oil and honey in a separate bowl and stir until combined. Put the bicarbonate of soda in a separate small bowl, add the boiling water and stir, then add to the honey and oil mixture and combine well.

Add the wet mixture to the dry ingredients and stir to combine well. Spread over the lined tray, flatten with your hands until even, then bake for 20 minutes or until melted and bubbling: don't worry if the mixture looks saucy, because once cooled it will become crunchy and sticky. Remove from the oven and allow to cool on the tray, then break into rough pieces or shards. Store in an airtight container for up to 10 days.

+ **NOTE** Wattleseed is a low glycaemic index (GI) food that releases energy slowly.

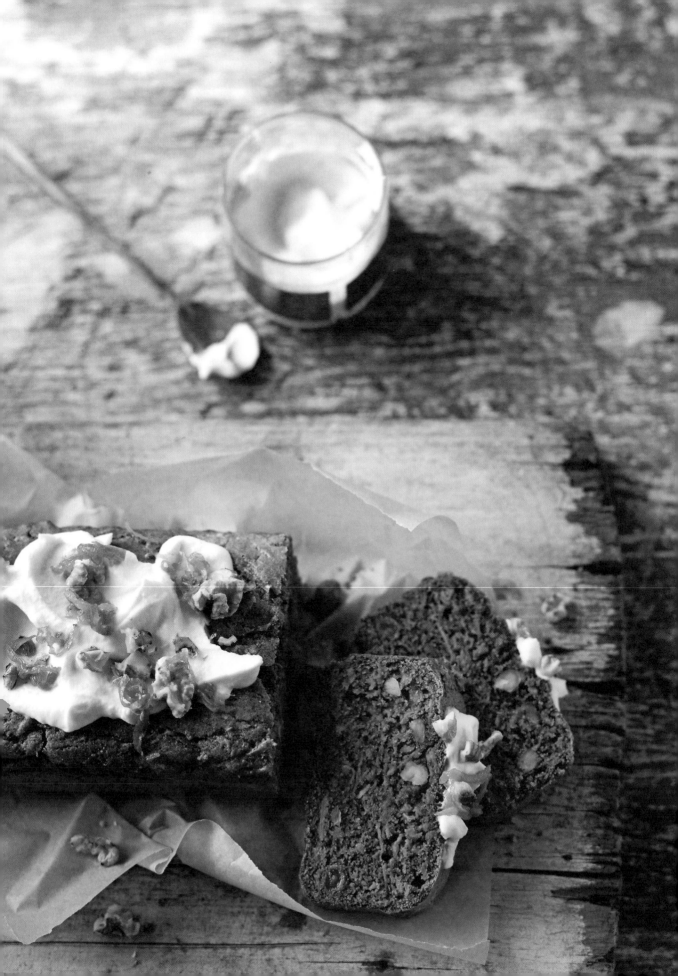

PREP TIME:
*30 minutes, plus
1 hour cooling*

COOKING TIME:
40 minutes

BEST-EVER CARROT & ZUCCHINI CAKE WITH RICOTTA FROSTING

The creamy topping is light but full of flavour.

SERVES 6–8

DRY MIX
100 g (3½ oz/1 cup) oat flour
80 g (2¾ oz/½ cup) green banana flour
1 teaspoon baking powder
½ teaspoon bicarbonate of soda (baking soda)
¼ teaspoon freshly grated nutmeg
2 teaspoons ground cinnamon
1 teaspoon ground ginger
½ teaspoon ground cloves
85 g (3 oz/½ cup) raisins
60 g (2½ oz/½ cup) chopped walnuts

WET MIX
2 large carrots, grated (about 2 cups)
1 large zucchini (courgette), grated (about 1 cup)
75 g (2¾ oz/½ cup) rapadura (unrefined cane sugar)
125 ml (4 fl oz/½ cup) olive oil
¼ teaspoon salt
3 eggs

TOPPING
1 tablespoon grated fresh ginger
½ small carrot, grated (about ¼ cup)
1 tablespoon honey
250 g (9 oz) ricotta cheese
30 g (1 oz/¼ cup) toasted walnuts

Preheat the oven to 160°C (315°F). Lightly grease a 30 x 12 x 10 cm (12 x 4½ x 4 inch) loaf (bar) tin and line it with baking paper, leaving the sides overhanging.

Put all of the dry mix ingredients in a large mixing bowl and stir to combine well. Put all of the wet mix ingredients in another bowl and whisk to combine well. Pour the wet ingredients into the dry mix and stir until well combined. Pour into the prepared tin and bake for 40 minutes or until a skewer comes out clean. Remove from the oven, allow to cool in the tin for 5 minutes, then remove and place on a wire rack to cool completely.

Meanwhile, put the ginger, carrot and honey in a frying pan over medium heat and stir for 5 minutes or until golden and sticky. Remove from the heat and allow to cool.

Put the ricotta in a bowl and beat with a wooden spoon until smooth. Spread over the cooled cake, then drizzle the ginger, honey and carrot mixture over the top. Scatter with chopped toasted walnuts and serve.

This cake will keep for up to 4 days in an airtight container.

+ **NOTE** I used green banana flour, which is simply ground green banana. It has a low glycaemic index (GI) with resistant starch that helps to create a great environment in your gut for good health.

PREP TIME:
25 minutes

COOKING TIME:
25 minutes

QUINOA SCONES

Indigenous Australians use the leaves of lemon myrtle for both hydration and a boost of nutrients.

MAKES 16 SCONES

DRY MIX
100 g (3½ oz/1 cup) quinoa flakes
120 g (4¼ oz/1 cup) quinoa flour
200 g (7 oz/2 cups) almond meal
30 g (1 oz/¼ cup) tapioca flour
2 teaspoons baking powder
½ teaspoon salt
2 tablespoons chia seeds
80 g (2¾ oz) unsalted butter,
    chilled and chopped

WET MIX
100 g (3½ oz/½ cup) coconut sugar
125 ml (4 fl oz/½ cup) tinned
    coconut milk
1 teaspoon lemon juice
2 eggs

LEMON MYRTLE YOGHURT
390 g (13¾ oz/1½ cups) Greek-style
    yoghurt
1 tablespoon ground lemon myrtle
Zest of 1 lemon

RASPBERRY CHIA JAM
125 g (4½ oz/1 cup) fresh or frozen
    raspberries
50 g (1¾ oz/¼ cup) coconut sugar
2 tablespoons coconut water
45 g (1½ oz/¼ cup) chia seeds

Preheat the oven to 160°C (315°F). Line a lightly greased baking tray with baking paper.

Put all of the ingredients for the dry mix, except the butter, in a mixing bowl and combine well. Using your fingertips, rub the butter into the dry ingredients until the mixture resembles coarse breadcrumbs.

Put all of the ingredients for the wet mix into a bowl. Add 2 tablespoons of water and use a hand-held whisk to beat until pale. Add to the dry mix and stir until the dough comes together, then transfer to a lightly floured work surface and knead for 4–5 minutes until smooth. Divide the mixture into 16 pieces, roll into balls and place on the prepared tray. Flatten slightly, then bake for 20–25 minutes until golden. Remove from the oven and allow to cool on the tray.

Meanwhile, to make the lemon myrtle yoghurt, put all of the ingredients in a small bowl and stir until well combined. Refrigerate until needed.

To make the raspberry chia jam, put all of the ingredients in a blender and process until the mixture thickens: the chia seeds will absorb most of the liquid, taking on a jelly-like texture.

Serve the cooled scones with the jam and lemon myrtle yoghurt. Scones are best served on the day of making.

+ GLUTEN-FREE
+ DAIRY-FREE
+ PALEO

PREP TIME:
10 minutes, plus
3 hours setting

COOKING TIME:
10 minutes

ALOE VERA SUMMER FRUIT TERRINE

*This recipe is great for the hotter months
as a lighter dessert for a dinner party.*

SERVES 6–8

1 litre (35 fl oz/4 cups) freshly
    squeezed apple juice
55 g (2 oz/⅓ cup) grass-fed bovine
    gelatine powder
80 ml (2½ fl oz/⅓ cup) aloe vera
    juice
80 g (2¾ oz/⅓ cup) frozen
    blackberries
60 g (2¼ oz/⅓ cup) frozen
    blueberries
70 g (2½ oz/⅓ cup) frozen
    strawberries
80 g (2¾ oz/⅓ cup) frozen
    raspberries
450 g (1 lb/2 cups) frozen mango
Mint leaves, to serve

Lightly grease a 30 x 12 x 10 cm (12 x 4½ x 4 inch) loaf (bar) tin and line it with plastic wrap, leaving the sides overhanging.

Combine 250 ml (9 fl oz/1 cup) of the apple juice and the gelatine in a bowl and stir to combine well.

Put the remaining apple juice in a saucepan over medium heat until close to boiling. Whisk in the gelatine mixture until well combined. Stir in the aloe vera juice and remove from the heat. Pour the mixture into the prepared tin and layer the fruit evenly over the jelly. Refrigerate for 3 hours or until set.

To serve, invert the terrine onto a serving dish, then scatter with mint leaves and serve.

+ **NOTE** Aloe vera juice is extracted from the leaves of this very useful plant. It's great for a healthy gut.

WHOLEFOODS ENTERTAINING: CHEESE BOARD

When I go back to basics, I choose cheese. Cheese and bread have been here for centuries and they are both made by a fermentation process that is full of good bacteria. I am the kind of girl who loves a cheese platter at the end of the meal or before — I just LOVE cheese!

SERVES 6

150 g (5½ oz) goat's cheddar
150 g (5½ oz) soft goat's cheese
100 g (3½ oz) roquefort (blue) cheese
200 g (7 oz) double-cream brie
120 g (4¼ oz) gruyère cheese
200 g (7 oz/1 cup) Peruvian groundcherries (Inca berries)
155 g (5½ oz/1 cup) Zesty Macadamias (see page 199)
180 g (6¼ oz/1 cup) grapes, fresh or muscatelles
165 g (5¾ oz/½ cup) Baobab & Orange Chia Jam (see page 67)
60 ml (2 fl oz/¼ cup) truffle oil
½ cup Matcha Dukkah (see page 112)
1 quantity Superfood Crackers (see page 200)
Sourdough bread, to serve

Remove all the cheeses from the fridge at least 30 minutes before serving: the longer the better.

Assemble all the cheeses on a platter. Scatter the berries, nuts and grapes around the cheese. Serve the remaining ingredients in small bowls with the crackers and bread on the side.

+ **NOTE** There is a great mantra for selecting cheese: "something old, something new, something goat, something blue". When eating cheese, the rule is to start with the mildest and work your way up to the strongest. Also make sure you choose good quality, locally made cheese to support your dairy farmers.

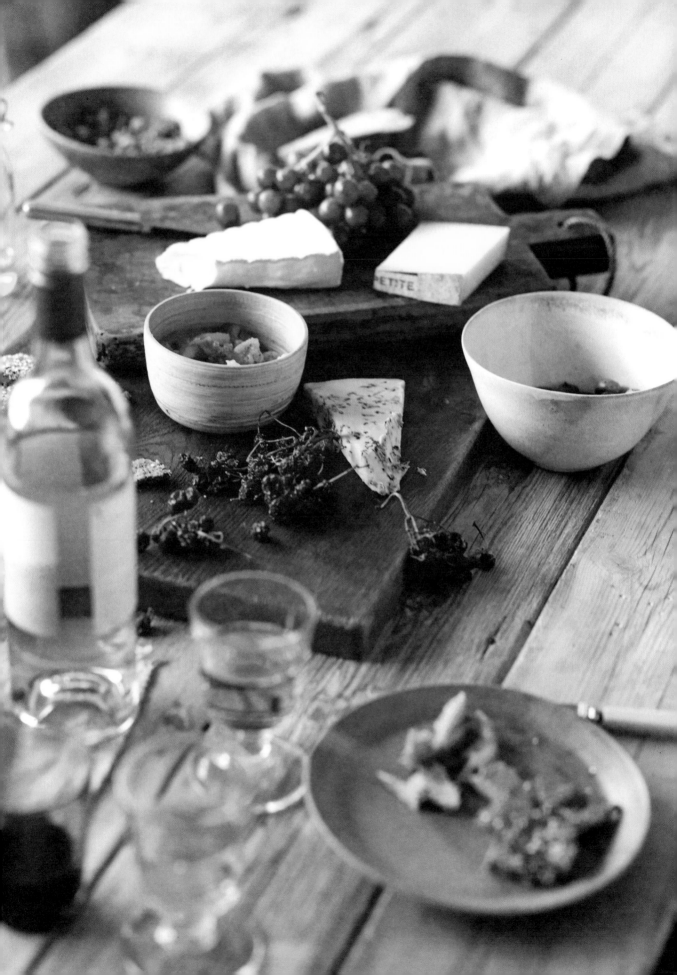

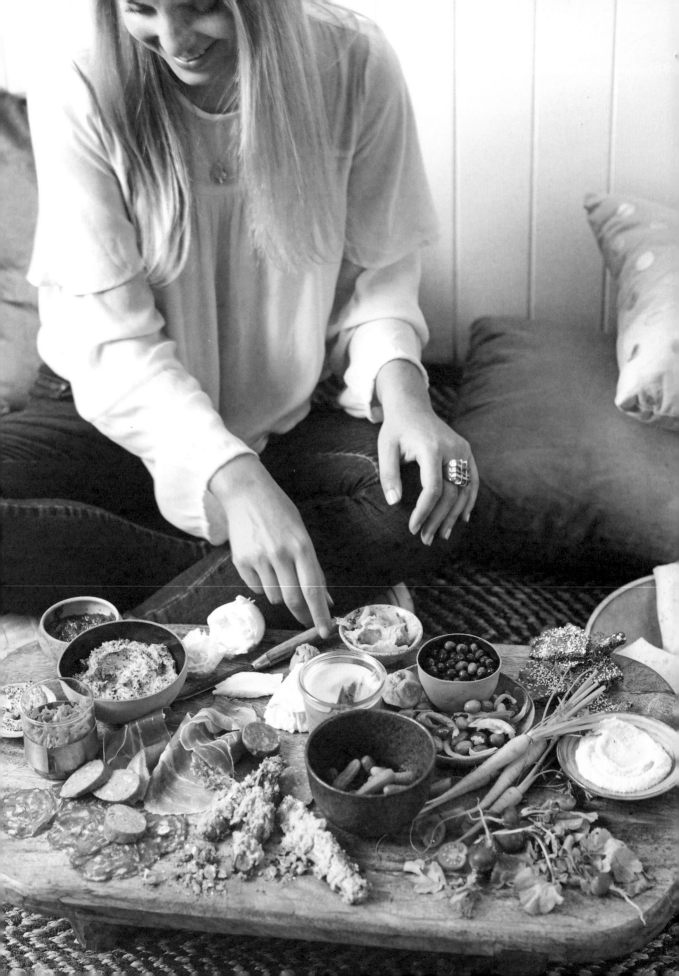

WHOLEFOODS ENTERTAINING: ANTIPASTO BOARD

I absolutely love creating an entertaining board. Here are some of my ideas for inspiration: it only takes 20 minutes to assemble, but I love taking my time with a glass of crisp wine.

SERVES 8

6 slices prosciutto
300 g (10½ oz) chorizo, sliced
16 slices salami
120 g (4¼ oz) pâté
300 g (10½ oz) olives
200 g (7 oz) buffalo mozzarella
150 g (5½ oz) goat's cheese
½ cup Pickled Veg (see page 173)
½ cup Pickled Kimchi (see page 171)
300 g (10½ oz) cornichons or
    dill gherkins
250 g (9 oz) cherry tomatoes
Selection of crudités
100 g (3½ oz) wholegrain mustard
Baked Eggplant Chips
    (see page 197)
Chia Olive Tapenade (see page 56)
250 g (9 oz/1 cup) Activated Raw
    Kale Pesto (see page 60)
220 g (7¾ oz/1 cup) Raw Nut
    Hummus (see page 65)
Superfood Crackers (see page 200)
125 ml (4 fl oz/½ cup) extra virgin
    olive oil
½ cup Matcha Dukkah
    (see page 112)
Bread, torn apart

Assemble all the ingredients on a big wooden board. Place the dips in little dishes, and the crudités and chips in separate jars. Serve with friends and lots of fun!

———

+ **NOTE** I have used little digestive dishes on this board, including kimchi, pickled vegies and cornichons, to get the digestion going.

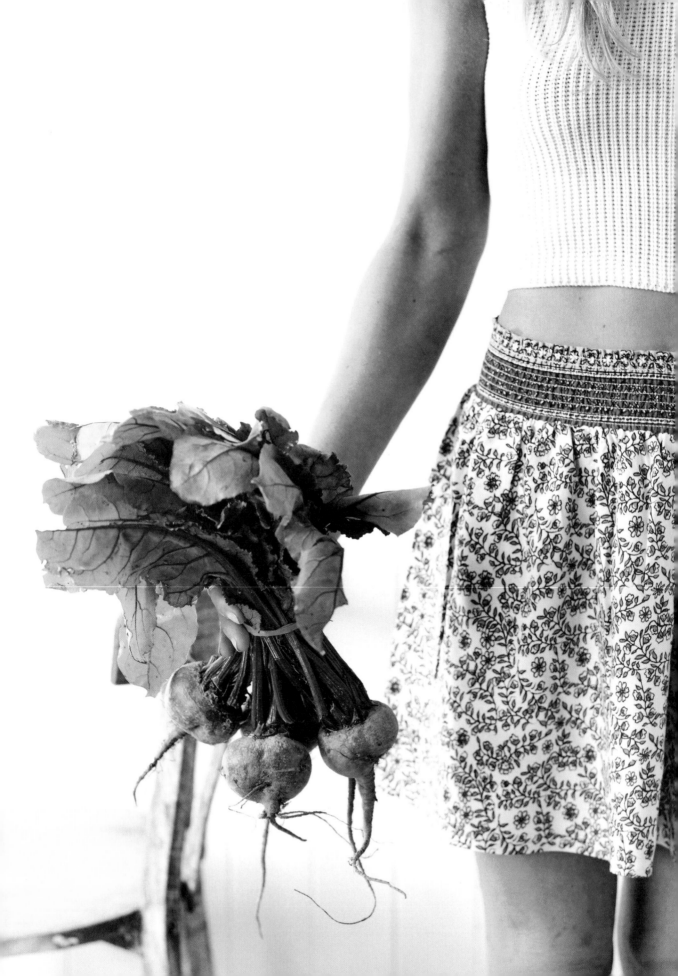

ACKNOWLEDGMENTS

My thanks to all who were part of this creation during amazing and crazy times – opening three stores in three months, at the same time as writing a cookbook, creating and testing all the recipes. I really could not have done this without support from so many.

Firstly I want to acknowledge the efforts of my amazing sister, Sandra, and my best friend and – lucky for me – colleague Pam, both of whom have worked endlessly on this project with me, making sure that I succeed. Thank you for putting up with me: I owe you big time! Also thank you to my family, so far away geographically in Slovakia, but so close to me every day when I think of you: I am grateful for Mami Lubica, Babi Jozephina, Nina, Ferko and Tati.

Thank you to Tammie and Jodie, the founders of About Life: inspiring sisters who get up every day and inspire not only me but everyone else in the About Life family. Their fierce passion and hard work is contagious.

My work is a joy every day and there is never a dull moment in this family.

I have so many people to be thankful to, from recipe testers to stylists to word wizards. Thank you particularly to Jonathan, Maggie, Sanna, Brano, Pepa, Rob, Alex, Giulia, Jane, Emily, Jennifer and Jean who navigated all of this. To the About Life team who all, in some way or another, have added to this book even without knowing it. It is so great to be part of such a great dynamic team. Cheers to us all!

Thanks too must go to the About Life customers who have supported me for so many years now and from whom I learn so much every day.

A special thank you to the whole Murdoch team: Jane and Hugh, Emma, Christine, Sarah, Melody, Michelle and Rob.

And lastly to all the dedicated farmers and producers who choose to work ethically and so very hard to supply us with the best quality produce – in its most natural state – that this planet has to offer.

INDEX

Published in 2017 by Murdoch Books, an imprint of Allen & Unwin

Murdoch Books Australia
83 Alexander Street
Crows Nest NSW 2065
Phone: +61 (0) 2 8425 0100
Fax: +61 (0) 2 9906 2218
murdochbooks.com.au
info@murdochbooks.com.au

Murdoch Books UK
Ormond House
26–27 Boswell Street
London WC1N 3JZ
Phone: +44 (0) 20 8785 5995
murdochbooks.co.uk
info@murdochbooks.co.uk

For Corporate Orders & Custom Publishing, contact
our Business Development Team at
salesenquiries@murdochbooks.com.au.

Publisher: Jane Morrow
Editorial Manager: Emma Hutchinson
Design Manager: Hugh Ford
Project Editor: Melody Lord
Designer: Sarah Odgers
Photographer: Rob Palmer
Stylist: Michelle Noerianto
Food Editor: Christine Osmond
Production Manager: Rachel Walsh

A cataloguing-in-publication entry is available from
the catalogue of the National Library of Australia
at nla.gov.au.

ISBN 978 1 74336 897 8 Australia
ISBN 978 1 74336 898 5 UK

A catalogue record for this book is available from the
British Library.

Colour reproduction by Splitting Image Colour Studio
Pty Ltd, Clayton, Victoria

Printed by 1010 Printing International Limited, China

IMPORTANT: Those who might be at risk from the
effects of salmonella poisoning or botulism (the elderly,
pregnant women, young children and those suffering
from immune deficiency diseases) should consult their
doctor with any concerns about eating raw eggs and
raw honey.

OVEN GUIDE: You may find cooking times vary
depending on the oven you are using. For fan-forced
ovens, as a general rule, set the oven temperature to
20°C (70°F) lower than indicated in the recipe.

MEASURES GUIDE: We have used 20 ml (4 teaspoon)
tablespoon measures. If you are using a 15 ml
(3 teaspoon) tablespoon add an extra teaspoon
of the ingredient for each tablespoon specified.